QR
182
.N53
1985

Nicholas, Robin.

Immunology, an
    information profile

DATE		

Immunology

An information profile

Robin and David Nicholas

Mansell Publishing Limited
London and New York

To Ashley and Thomas Nicholas

First published 1985 by Mansell Publishing Limited
(A subsidiary of The H. W. Wilson Company)
6 All Saints Street, London N1 9RL, England
950 University Avenue, Bronx, New York 10452, U.S.A.

British Library Cataloguing in Publication Data

Nicholas, Robin
  Immunology: an information profile.
  1. Immunology — Information services
  2. Immunology — Bibliography
  I. Title   II. Nicholas, D. (David), *1947*–
  574.2′9   QR181

ISBN 0-7201-1724-0

Library of Congress Cataloging in Publication Data

Nicholas, Robin
  Immunology: an information profile.

  Bibliography: p.
  Includes index.
  1. Immunology — Information services.
  I. Nicholas, David. II. Title. [DNLM: 1. Allergy and Immunology.
  2. Allergy and Immunology — bibliography.
  3. Information Services.   QW 504 N599i]
QR182.N53   1985   616.07′9′072   84-21773
ISBN 0-7201-1724-0 (U.S.)

Printed in Great Britain by
Henry Ling Ltd., at the Dorset Press, Dorchester, Dorset

Contents

Preface

Immunology is undeniably the fastest-growing and most 'popular' of the biological sciences. Evidence for this is widespread; the number of immunology journals is growing exponentially and now stands at over 80, and is increasing at 5 a year; the number of national immunology societies has increased threefold since 1970; the number of jobs advertised for posts requiring immunological skills has increased enormously, largely as a result of the great commercial interest shown in biotechnology; and the number of meetings locally and worldwide devoted to immunological topics has multiplied.

Why has there been this upsurge in interest in an area which is concerned chiefly with the activities of only one kind of cell, the lymphocyte, and its secretory products, which mainly comprise the antibody?

There is of course no simple answer. J. H. Humphrey, writing in *The Biologist* (1980), attributes the success of immunology to various factors. Antibodies have proved to be useful tools in other disciplines; advances in immunology have provided cheap and effective ways to combat disease; there is the fascinating question immunology poses of how, at the cellular level, an individual distinguishes 'self' from 'non-self'; and immunology has ensured the ready availability of lymphocytes and antibodies.

Whilst these reasons are of course important, there are others, the most important of which is that immunological research can prove to be a wise financial investment. In these terms the major money spinner undoubtedly is hybridoma technology, and its chief product the monoclonal antibody. The central role immunology has played in the development of molecular biology in general, and recombinant DNA technology in particular, is also part of the field's success story. Finally one should not ignore the fact that the production of vaccines against infectious diseases is still the main motivating force behind immunology.

The problems confronted by those seeking information on immunology are indeed enormous. The major problem is really that of scale; so much is going on, on such a wide front, and in such a short space of time, that few can hope to keep track of what is going on (never mind digest much of it), or effectively retrieve information from a rapidly shifting and expanding information archive. And it is not as if researchers can walk away from the information problem, as they may in other fields, for here the penalties of ignorance can be great, both in scientific and commercial terms.

Yet information tools do exist which provide some measure of control, and multiple access to research output, but they have proliferated so greatly, and are of such large size (most embrace either the whole literature of biology, medicine or biotechnology), that there is a real danger of information getting in the way of information.

Despite the advent of online technology (to which this book addresses itself in some detail), and its ability to take the drudgery out of searching vast banks of data, the ideal solution for the beleaguered scientist — a one-place reference for all his information needs — is still seemingly a long way off. So, to keep in touch with what is going on in the field, the researcher will inevitably have to consult numerous and varied sources, though the fact that he can access many of them through just one computer terminal, which may be conveniently located by his desk, does make the search somewhat more bearable, and perhaps a little more pleasurable.

The function of this book is a simple one: it is to make known to those seeking immunological information those information sources that aim to provide for the everyday information needs of immunologists. By doing this we hope to provide a one-place reference to all sources of immunological information, regardless of the disciplines they originate from. An additional purpose is to suggest how immunologists may keep abreast of the new information tools and developments to come.

The guide is mainly limited to English-language sources, basically for practical reasons: our experience of foreign-language sources is limited and many of them are inaccessible. Furthermore the sheer size of the task means that some degree of selection is necessary, and it seemed appropriate to draw the boundary along these lines, particularly as the most important sources are in English anyway. As many of the sources dealt with are international in scope, and are used as widely in Europe as in the United States, we feel that we have not wholly neglected foreign-language materials.

It is hoped that this work will provide, albeit for a relatively short space of time, the coherence and structure that is so patently lacking from the literature of immunology. The profile has been designed as a self-help tool, and as such addresses itself to those with little formal knowledge of either information sources or indeed immunology itself.

Acknowledgements

Special thanks go to Chris and Kay Nicholas for typing the manuscript and for their many useful suggestions.

We would also like to thank the International Union of Immunological Societies and the British Society for Immunology for providing some useful documents; the staff of the Central Veterinary Laboratory's library for their prompt and efficient service; and Nick Reed for help with some of the figures.

Some abbreviations used in this book

AACIA	American Association for Clinical Immunology and Allergy
AAI	American Association of Immunologists
AFRC	Agricultural and Food Research Council
AIDS	Acquired immune deficiency syndrome
B-cell	B-lymphocyte
BSI	British Society of Immunology
CIOMS	Council for International Organizations of Medical Sciences
ECCLS	European Committee for Clinical Laboratory Standards
EFIS	European Federation of Immunological Societies
ELISA	Enzyme-linked immunosorbent assay
EMBO	European Molecular Biology Organization
FASEB	Federation of American Societies for Experimental Biology
HLA	Human leukocyte antigen
IAA	International Association of Allergology
ICSU	International Council of Scientific Unions
ISDCI	International Society of Developmental and Comparative Immunology
IUIS	International Union of Immunological Societies
IUMS	International Union of Microbiological Societies
LCM	Lymphocytic choriomeningitis
MAFF	Ministry of Agriculture, Fisheries and Food
MCA or Mabs	Monoclonal antibody
MCH	Major histocompatibility complex
MRC	Medical Research Council
NCCLS	National Committee for Clinical Laboratory Standards
NCI	National Cancer Institute
NIAID	National Institute of Allergy and Infectious Diseases
NIBSC	National Institute for Biological Standardization and Control
NIH	National Institutes of Health
NK cells	Natural killer cells
PHLS	Public Health Laboratory Service
RES	Reticulo-endothelial Society
SLE	Systemic lupus erythematosus
T-cell	T-lymphocyte
WAVMI	World Association of Veterinary Microbiologists, Immunologists and Specialists in Infectious Diseases
WHO	World Health Organization

Part 1

OVERVIEW OF IMMUNOLOGY AND ITS LITERATURE

1 Immunology: the subject

1.1 HISTORY AND DEVELOPMENT

For immunology, the meeting which took place in Washington, D.C., in the first week of August 1971 represented a major milestone in its development as an independent scientific discipline. The meeting, the First International Congress of Immunology, attracted most of the world's leading immunologists, numbering some 3500, from 45 countries. Not only were the quantity and quality of delegates a feature of this historic gathering, but also the timing, for such had been the breathtakingly rapid progress of research in the subject that all the most important conceptual questions appeared for the first time to be answerable.

Immunology had arrived, but when and what were its origins?

Traditionally, immunology's roots are traced to the late eighteenth century when Edward Jenner, a physician from south-west England, exploited a common observation that dairy workers who were exposed to cowpox, a relatively harmless disease in humans, were by and large resistant to smallpox. Jenner deliberately induced cowpox in his human subjects with material from diseased cattle; then, after a suitable interval, infected them with smallpox to see whether they were protected; in most cases they were. In 1798 Jenner published his work in a modest pamphlet entitled: 'An enquiry into the causes and effects of variolae vaccinae, a disease, discovered in some of the western counties of England, particularly Gloucestershire, and known by the name of cowpox' (a title that would not have got past most modern publishers!).

Jennerian vaccination, as it came to be called, dominated the scene for the next hundred years and certainly laid the basis for modern immunization practises. But in fact the concept was not startlingly new; it had been known since ancient Greek times that people who recovered from some infectious diseases did not succumb again to the same infection.

The Chinese, then later the Turks, practised 'variolation' whereby patients were inoculated with a, hopefully, mild smallpox infection. Lady Wortley-Montague introduced this practice into England at around 1720, and while it may appear hazardous, not to say desperate, to our eyes, variolation was the major factor in the population explosion which began during the first half of the eighteenth century.

Important as he was, Jenner has not been recognized as the founding father of immunology because his work was largely empirical, and he did not know how vaccination actually worked. Instead it was Louis Pasteur who, pondering on the obvious success of Jennerian vaccination, intentionally and thoughtfully attenuated fowl cholera cultures and showed that such cultures could induce immunity, could claim the mantle of immunology's founding father. The year now recognized as the birth of immunology is 1880, when Pasteur began his experimental work on disease prevention. With fowl cholera the underlying principle was that aged cultures lose their virulence (i.e. become attenuated) but retain the capacity to induce immunity.

Within a few months Pasteur had discovered the same phenomenon in veterinary anthrax, and successfully developed a vaccine against the disease. But the most dramatic of Pasteur's work involved the human disease hydrophobia, or rabies. Attenuation of the causative agent, a virus in this case, was achieved by drying spinal cords from infected rabbits. A vaccine prepared from the spinal cords was, after successful animal experimentation, shown to be effective in saving the life of a boy who had received multiple bites from a rabid dog.

The age of bacteriology

The years 1880 to approximately 1910 were a period of great activity and high hopes. This period came to be known as the 'age of bacteriology' because most of the immunological research was taking place in bacteriological laboratories on, chiefly, bacterial diseases. In 1886 Salmon and Theobold-Smith demonstrated that heat-killed cultures of fowl cholera were also effective in protecting birds from infection, thus alleviating the risk of relying on attenuated organisms that could spontaneously revert and show an enhanced degree of virulence. Roux and Yersin, in 1888, discovered that a bacterium-free filtrate of a culture of the diphtheria bacillus contained a toxin which could evoke a specific neutralizing substance, or antitoxin, in the blood of an immune animal, and that by means of such antitoxin immunity could be transferred from one animal to another. This result was first recorded in the case of tetanus antitoxin by Von Behring and Kitasato in 1890. It was shown that not only toxins but all sorts of materials including snake venom and ricin — a poisonous extract from castor oil — could elicit neutralizing substances generally called antibodies. Other properties attaching to antibodies were discovered: bacteriolysis (by Pfeiffer and Issaef in 1894); precipitation (Kraus, 1897); and agglutination (Gruber and Durham, 1898). These reactions were all specific: the antibodies in the immune sera reacted only with the material (or antigen as the inoculating agent came to be called) that evoked them. Thus these 'serological' reactions could be used to detect the presence of disease-causing organisms in the blood of patients. Furthermore the knowledge acquired opened up the possibility of serotherapy, whereby patients suffering from infectious diseases such as diphtheria could be given the serum of an immunized animal, as first shown by Roux in 1894. Unfortunately in no case was serum ever found to act as dramatically as in diphtheria. However, interest in serotherapy led to further knowledge of the immunological properties of immune serum, most important of which was the discovery of a heat-sensitive constituent, later called complement, which had bactericidal action (Buchner, 1893).

As immunologists became aware of the exquisite specificity of antibodies they were soon using it to analyse the antigenic make-up of bacteria and other antigenic complexes. In 1900 Karl Landsteiner, who was to become very important in the field, used natural antisera to recognize the different antigenic components in the red blood cells — the A, B, and O blood groups. Also in the same year Nuttall, Wasserman and Schultze reported that they could distinguish human, cow's and goat's milk by using the precipitation test.

So far attention had been directed solely on the constituents of immune serum — the so-called humoral factors — for the basis of the immune reaction to infectious disease. This was to change, and with the change came the first of many, at times violent, controversies which racked the discipline.

Eli Metchnitoff, a Russian, was convinced that the most important factor lay in the ability of certain cells, the leukocytes, to ingest and destroy microorganisms by a process called phagocytosis. The resulting dispute between advocates of antibodies, mainly the Germans, and Metchnikoff and his 'cellular immunologists' was however reconciled by the findings of Wright and Denys in 1903 that certain serum factors facilitated phagocytosis.

While discoveries were coming thick and fast, what was still fundamentally lacking was a theoretical framework in which to work. Paul Ehrlich put forward a general theory of immunity in 1897 under the name of the 'side chain' or 'receptor' theory in which antigen and antibody combined chemically in fixed proportions and with a discrete and absolute specificity. It had a profound influence in stimulating fundamental work on the mechanism of antibody production. It also had a profound effect on the Belgian immunologist Jules Bordet, who opposed it vehemently! Bordet's contention was that antibody combined in varying proportions. Thus began the famous Ehrlich–Bordet debates; the chemist versus the biologist. Proof that Ehrlich's concept was closer to the truth did not come for fifty years. For their efforts both received a Nobel Prize – Ehrlich in 1909 (shared incidentally with Metchnikoff) and Bordet in 1919.

While the dispute between Ehrlich and Bordet was marked by politeness and respect, the same could not be said for the 'debate' which took place between Ehrlich and Max von Gruber at around the same time. Without going into the details of the nature of their dispute, save for the fact that Gruber believed a single antibody could interact by graded affinities with a number of different antigens, the conflict between the protagonists was certainly personal, vitriolic and, at times, incomprehensible since each spoke a different language.

If the excitement of these early years was not enough, the next event to occur was highly unexpected. It was observed, initially by Portier and Richet (1902), then later by Arthus (1903), that reinjection of even bland antigens into immunized animals could produce severe symptoms, even death, a condition known as anaphylaxis. (The term 'allergy', first coined by von Pirquet (1906) was later generalized to include all sensitization phenomena.) The widely held view that antibodies were designed specifically to protect the host had received a major setback. It now appeared that the immunological response could, under certain states of 'hypersensitivity', result in damage to the host's own cells; the cause of this was thought to be histamine (Dale and Laidlaw, 1910).

The first three decades of this new, independent branch of medical science witnessed the discovery and description of most of the fundamental immunological phenomena. The closing stages of this period saw the publication in Germany of the very first journal devoted to immunology, entitled *Zeitschrift fuer Immunitaetsforschung*, in 1909: further proof, if it was needed, that immunology was emerging as a self-sustaining discipline. (This journal is now known as *Immunobiology (Stuttgart) Zeitschrift für Immunitätsforschung*.) Just seven years later the newly founded American Association of Immunologists began publication of the *Journal of Immunology*, which soon became the leading vehicle for immunological research, a position it has maintained throughout its 70 years of existence.

Prior to the publication of these two immunology journals, research into the nature of immunity had been scattered throughout a variety of medical journals: *Journal of Experimental Medicine, Journal of Infectious Diseases, Journal of Medical Research, Proceedings of the Society for Experimental Biology and Medicine* and *Proceedings of the Royal Society of London* were the major English-language journals. In addition, much information lay in the more obscure (at least from a British and American standpoint) foreign-language journals, the most important of which were the *Wiener Klinische Wochenschrift*, the *Münchener Medizinische Wochenschrift*, the *Berliner Klinische Wochenschrift, Annales de l'Institut Pasteur* and *Zentralblatt für Bakteriologie*.

The most important books of the period were, like the journals, mostly written in German or French: *L'Immunité dans les maladies infectieuses* was the title given to two original works, one by Achalme (1895) and the other by Metchnikoff (1901); and *Immunität und Immunisierung*, another classic, was written by Hope in 1902. Fortunately for English-speaking immunologists the publishers translated the works by Ehrlich (1906) and Bordet (1909), both entitled *Studies in immunity*. *Immunochemistry* by Arrhenius (1907), another important text, was translated and published in New York.

The predominance of books and journals published in German and French was of course an accurate reflection of the enormous amount of work being carried out on the Continent. Indeed Vienna in the 1890s certainly had claim to being the intellectual and scientific centre of Europe, if not the world. For immunology, the epicentre was the newly established Department of Hygiene at the University of Vienna, where Landsteiner (often referred to as 'the complete immunologist') and his mentor Von Gruber were to make such an impact on the field. In Paris the Institut Pasteur, founded in 1880 and led by Louis Pasteur himself until his death in 1895, attracted many of the leading immunologists of the day: Roux, Yersin, and later Metchnikoff. Bordet, too, began his work at the Institut Pasteur in Paris in 1894 before helping to set up the Institut Pasteur in Brussels in 1900. Koch's Institute for Infectious Disease in Berlin was the scene of Von Behring and Kitasato's antitoxin work, as well as much of the research carried out by Ehrlich. Von Behring was particularly active at the time; he was associated with the Royal Prussian Institute for Experimental Therapy, and gave his name to the Behring Institute in Marburg (1893).

Undoubtedly then, the most significant debates and contributions were coming from Continental Europe. However with the defeat and dissolution of the Austro-Hungarian empire and, following shortly on its heels, the defeat of the Axis Powers in the First World War, the pendulum began to move west towards Britain and the USA — where in fact significant contributions had already been made. In the USA, for instance, the Johns Hopkins University School of Hygiene and Public Health could boast one of the world's first Departments of Immunology. Other important centres included Cornell University's Department of Experimental Medicine, Harvard University Medical School, the McManes Laboratory of Experimental Pathology at the University of Pennsylvania, and the Rockefeller Institute. The USA also started the first society devoted solely to the study of immunology — the American Society of Immunologists — which was founded in 1913, pre-dating the second immunological society by over 40 years. In Britain the Lister Institute, the London Hospital, University College, London, and the Medical Schools of Oxford and Cambridge were most active in immunology.

The age of immunochemistry

The phases which are assigned to the development of immunology between the years 1880 and the present day are of course artificial; the workers at the time were certainly not aware of moving from one period to another. But none the less it is interesting to try to identify particular trends that were occurring. With this in mind the years from around 1910 to the 1940s have come to be known as the 'age of immunochemistry'.

Immunology during this period was dominated by chemical approaches and chemical thinking. The titles of the leading books in immunology published at the time provided evidence of this: *The chemistry of antigens and antibodies* by J. R. Marrack (1934); *The chemical aspects in immunity* by H. G. Wells (1924); and *Quantitative immunochemistry* by E. A. Kabat and M. M. Mayer (1949). Immunology papers were beginning to appear in such chemical and biochemical journals as *Biochemisches Zeitschrift, Zeitschrift für Physiologische Chemie* and the *Journal of the American Chemical Society*.

Among the most productive applications of chemistry to immunology were the studies of the ubiquitous Landsteiner and his collaborators. After the First World War Landsteiner had lost his position in Vienna, and moved temporarily to the Netherlands, before finally accepting an invitation to take up a position at the Rockefeller Institute in New York, where his work flourished. He showed that the properties of antibodies could be altered by treating antigens with chemicals, and originated the term 'hapten' in 1921. Such work was to show the world the elegance and fine precision of immunological specificity, and he won a Nobel Prize in 1930 for this work. Landsteiner's book, *The specificity of serological reactions*, published in German in 1933 and in English in 1936, summarized his work, and greatly influenced the research of many others.

Michael Heidelberger, working at the University of Columbia, developed accurate quantitative methods for measuring the amounts of antibody in serum which could combine with a given antigen, and confirmed that when antigens were reinoculated into an animal months, or even years later, the specific antibody elicited appeared sooner and in much larger amounts than on the first occasion, showing that the animal had 'remembered' the antigen.

It seemed amazing that all this information had been acquired about the properties of antibodies, when it was not until 1939 that it was shown that antibodies were proteins belonging to the gamma-globulin class first identified in serum by Tiselius in 1937. This term immunoglobulin has come to be synonymous with antibodies.

In parallel with the developments in immunochemistry, some progress was being made, notably the confirmation of Pfeiffer and Marx's observation, in 1898, that the leukocytes manufacture antibodies. It was not until 1948 that Astrid Fagraeus showed that the actual synthesis of antibodies took place through the development of plasma cells. The 'decade of cellular immunology', which is how the 1970s are recognized, was still however a long way off.

Slow progress was also being made in the applied areas of immunology. Prophylactic vaccines were greatly improved and made safer, particularly after Ramon and Glenny, in 1923, were able to show that several toxin preparations could be detoxified by formaldehyde treatment without losing their ability to raise an immune response. The use of antitoxins to treat dangerous bacterial infections, such as pneumonia, tetanus and gas gangrene, also became more widespread. During the Second World War immunization was extended to cover a new range of diseases, such as dysentery and mumps.

This period also saw some important technical advances. The quantitative precipitation method described by Heidelberger and Kendall (1935) was the most important single factor in the development of modern immunochemistry, enabling antigens or antibodies to be detected, quantified and distinguished from others. Another important advance was Coons' (1942) use of specific antibodies, with a fluorescent label attached, to detect antigens or antibodies in single cells. Others included ultracentrifugation (Svedberg and Pederson, 1939), ultrafiltration through membranes (Elford, Grabar, 1930–35), electrophoresis in liquid medium (Tiselius, 1937) and filtration through absorption columns (Porath, 1950).

Surprisingly perhaps, the rapid developments on the laboratory bench were not being paralleled by growth in the number of journals reporting immunological research. Only two major publications, *Acta Allergologica* (later *Allergy*) and the *Journal of Allergy and Clinical Immunology*, appeared between 1920 and 1950. The early fifties produced *International Archives of Allergy and Applied Immunology*, the Italian *Folia Allergologica et Immunologica Clinica*, and the German *Allergie und Asthma* (later *Allergie und Immunologie*), and it was not until 1958 that the first British immunology journal, *Immunology*, appeared, which was published by the British Society for Immunology commencing two years after the Society was founded.

As immunology moved into the 1950s, the journals which carried most of the research findings were still the *Journal of Immunology* and the *Journal of Experimental Medicine;* there were also some biochemical ones such as *Biochimica et Biophysica Acta* and the *Biochemical Journal*.

The age of immunobiology

The 1950s and early 1960s have come to be regarded as 'the age of immunobiology' because they saw immunological research shift its emphasis towards biology. During these years the foundations of transplantation immunology, cancer immunology and immunopathology were laid. The period also provided for the first time a modern theoretical framework. In retrospect the first serious attempt can be seen to have been made in a monograph entitled *The production of antibody* by Burnet and Fenner in 1949, in which the authors argued that animals would not raise antibodies to antigens that they had come into contact with during fetal or early neonatal life — they would be regarded as 'self'. This provided an explanation as to why animals tolerated their own tissue, cells, etc., but would not tolerate the introduction of foreign material. In 1953 Medawar and colleagues confirmed the hypothesis experimentally. Then in 1959 Talmage, and Burnet and Lederberg, put forward a 'clonal selection hypothesis' to explain the biology of immune responses. In essence this stated that the immunologically responsive cell (guessed by Burnet to be a 'lymphocyte' — a rather featureless leukocyte) can respond to only one antigen, or a few related ones, and that this ability is somehow acquired before the antigen is met. On meeting the antigen the lymphocyte is stimulated to multiply and produce a clone of identical cells, some of which secrete antibody, while others circulate through the blood and tissues and act as 'memory cells'. The same antigen encountered by the 'memory' cells months or years later evokes a more rapid and copious secondary response.

In the same year Gowans published the first of a series of papers which proved that lymphocytes actually were the immunologically responsive cells. A year later Porter and Edelman elucidated the general structure of antibodies. It was now the turn of the molecular biologists and geneticists to make their contribution by revealing the secrets of the immune response at the biochemical level.

But where was the research work itself taking place? It was mentioned earlier that the centre of activity had moved westwards from Continental Europe to Britain and the USA, a process which received added impetus both before and during the Second World War. Significant contributions had also come from Australia, particularly from the John Curtin School of Medical Research at the Australian National University, and the Walter and Eliza Hall Institute for Medical Research. In Britain the National Institute for Medical Research, founded in the 1920s, played a leading role in pioneering immunological research. Other important laboratories included the Sir William Dunn School of Pathology at Oxford (later to house the Medical Research Council's Immunology Unit); University College, London; and the Clinical Research Centre, also in London. In the USA the universities, the main beneficiaries of the influx of immigrants from Europe, had begun to rise in eminence. Some have already been mentioned; others included Chicago, Rockefeller, Stanford and New York.

And, of course, there is Japan. Japanese effort was considerable but largely unseen because, for at least two decades until the 1970s, many Japanese scientists had worked abroad as postdoctoral fellows in immunology, particularly in the USA. On their return they began to improve the quality of research already taking place in laboratories like the Institute for Medical Sciences at Tokyo University, and the Kitasato Institute for Infectious Diseases (named after Von Behring's Japanese co-worker S. Kitasato).

The age of cellular immunology

The late 1960s and the 1970s were remarkable years for immunology. Up to this time immunological information had been scattered widely in medical journals and books, and immunologists' interests were shared with microbiologists, pathologists and others. Suddenly and rapidly it all changed. The instrument of change must surely have been the International Union of Immunological Societies (IUIS) which was founded in 1969. Initially representing some 10 national societies, it has since increased its membership to 33, with a few more shortly to be accepted. Just two years later the First International Congress was held in Washington, D.C. In the publishing field the number of journals devoted to immunology mushroomed from not much more than a dozen to the 80 or so published today; regular review volumes — a sure indication of considerable research activity — increased to nearly 30, and the number of monographs and books published climbed to the thousand mark. The explosion in the literature shows no signs of abating, many new journals and serials having been started in the 1980s. Many institutes and university departments of immunology have also been founded or renamed to include the word 'immunology', the most notable being the Basel Institute for Immunology, which became operational in 1971. It is entirely financed by Hoffman-La Roche but guaranteed full academic freedom.

In the area of research, activity had been equally intense. The 1970s were dubbed the 'decade of cellular immunology' because of the increasing interest in lymphocytes. It was discovered that there were essentially two main types: first, B-lymphocytes, which develop in the bursa in chickens (and elsewhere in mammals), and are chiefly responsible for secreting antibody; secondly, the T-lymphocytes, which develop in the thymus — like the B-lymphocyte these can recognize and respond to foreign antigens, but unlike B-lymphocytes they do not respond by secreting antibody. Instead T-lymphocytes have become recognized as the cells that regulate the behaviour of B-lymphocytes, and are responsible, either directly, or in co-operation with macrophages (the body's scavenger cells), for important aspects of the body's defences against invaders, particularly viruses. It also seems that they prevent the growth of some tumours. However they also provide the main impediment to successful organ transplantation from donors if donor and host are not perfectly matched.

Much more has been learnt about the structure, function and types of anti-bodies and lymphocytes, that is not only beyond the scope of this very general introduction but, in many aspects, beyond the comprehension of the present authors — such are the complexities of the immunological concepts and its vocabulary for anyone not at the cutting edge of research. Today the structure of the antibody molecule, and the location and nature of its combining sites, have been worked out in the finest detail. Paul Ehrlich's suggestion of 1897 that immunological specificity was based on a 'chemical' three-dimensional arrange-ment of atoms in the antibody molecule, that enabled close combination of the antigen, had been a brilliant conceptual leap for his times; over fifty years went by before it was verified.

Finally, two more momentous events occurred in the 1970s. The first has revolutionized not only immunology but many areas of the biomedical and agri-cultural sciences. It began with the publication of a paper in the journal *Nature* in 1975 entitled: 'Continuous cultures of fused cells secreting antibody of a predetermined specificity' by Georges Kohler and Cesar Milstein, working at the Laboratory of Molecular Biology at Cambridge. Briefly the key pivot of their work — the production of exactly similar (monoclonal) antibody molecules out-side the body — was the fusion of the antibody-producing lymphocyte (found mainly in the spleen of immunized animals) with a myeloma cell (a cancer cell which endows the normally short-lived lymphocyte with immortality). Thus it was possible for them to generate unlimited supplies of these hybrid cells which continuously produce monoclonal antibody of the specificity desired by the worker. Applications of hybridoma (the suffix -oma is borrowed from the collec-tivization of cancer cells) technology have been wide-ranging, particularly in clinical medicine where monoclonal antibodies are being used for passive immunization, the protection of grafted tissues and organs and the destruction of tumours. In the research laboratory they have been used for differentiating and purifying viruses and bacteria, characterizing antigens in cancer, and purifying interferons. The potential of monoclonal antibodies is therefore enormous — as is generally recognized by the financial community.

Finally, the second great event of the 1970s was the declaration by the World Health Organization in 1977 that smallpox had been eradicated, a situation that had been achieved by a policy of mass worldwide immunization using a vaccine not all that dissimilar from the one introduced by Edward Jenner nearly two hundred years before.

1.2 SCOPE, DEFINITION AND SUBJECT RELATIONSHIPS

The International Union of Immunological Societies identified three main areas which constitute the study of immunology: first, problems internal to immunology itself such as the structure of antibodies; secondly, biological problems linking immunology to other biosciences such as using immunological markers and methods for the study of cell membrane structure; and thirdly, areas of research which intrinsically have little to do with immunology but in which immunological methods significantly contribute to progress, such as the use of radio-immunological hormone assays in endocrinology.

In many ways the development of monoclonal antibodies has, more than any other factor, widened the scope of immunology; one use currently proposed is to use them to identify molecules that may be important as flavourings in the food industry. *Figure 1.1* shows the possible and actual applications of monoclonal antibodies in two important areas of medicine: diagnosis and control.

Most textbooks divide immunology into two areas, basic and clinical. Basic immunology is said to cover the structure, function and development of the cells, organs and molecules of the immune system. Clinical (quite literally 'at the sick bed') immunology includes immuno-deficiency diseases, autoimmunity, hypersensitivity and allergy, and transplantation.

Immunology may be divided more specifically into the following main areas of research, although these areas are not mutually exclusive and there is, inevitably, some overlapping:

1. Allergy: including hypersensitivity, and atopic diseases such as hay fever and asthma.
2. Autoimmunity: concerned with the situation where normal 'self' tolerance is not established, or where this breaks down with the production of auto-antibodies.
3. Cancer immunology: the study of tumour cell antigens; and the investigation of immunological diagnosis and control of tumours.
4. Cellular immunology: the study of the cells — lymphocytes — and organs involved in the immune response.
5. Immunochemistry: mainly concerned with technical aspects such as immunoassays and radio-labelling.
6. Immunogenetics: including the genetic control of the immune response.
7. Immunohaematology: mainly concerned with the different blood groups, and disorders.
8. Immunopathology: studies organ damage by immune complexes.
9. Microbial immunology (immunoparasitology): the study of antigens of bacteria, viruses and parasites; development of vaccines.
10. Molecular immunology: the study of the chemical structure of antigens and antibodies; also includes the analysis of complement.

Table 1.1 Milestones in immunology

1720	Lady Wortley-Montague introduces 'variolation' to Britain
1798	Jenner practises vaccination against smallpox
1880	The birth of immunology proper — Pasteur attenuates fowl cholera
1881–5	Pasteur vaccinates against rabies and anthrax
1882	Metchnikoff expounds cellular immunology
1888	Roux and Yersin discover diphtheria antitoxin
1890	Von Behring and Kitasato describe tetanus antitoxin
1893	Buchner discovers complement
1894	Roux practises serotherapy against diphtheria
1897	Ehrlich's 'side chain' theory
1900	Landsteiner distinguishes blood groups
1902	Portier and Richet describe anaphylaxis
1903	Wright and Denys report serum factors, 'opsonins', capable of enhancing phagocytosis
1906	Von Pirquet coins the term 'allergy'
1909	First journal of immunology: *Zeitschrift fuer Immunitaetsforschung*
1910	Dale and Laidlow report histamine's involvement in immunological responses
1913	American Association of Immunologists founded
1916	Immunology's premier journal, *Journal of Immunology*, founded
1921	Landsteiner describes the properties of 'haptens'
1923	Ramon and Glenny detoxify by formaldehyde treatment
1935	Landsteiner and Kendall introduce quantitative precipitation method
1938	Tiselius and Kabat identify antibodies as gamma-globulins
1943	Chase transfers delayed hypersensitivity by use of lymphocytes
1944	Medawar shows that skin graft rejection is an immune response
1949	Burnet and Fenner publish *The production of antibody*
1953	Billingham, Brent and Medawar show 'self tolerance'
1956	Roitt and Doniach describe thyroid disease auto-antibodies
1956	British Society for Immunology founded
1959	Burnet, Lederberg and Talmage expounded their clonal selection theory
1959	Gowans confirms the immunological responsiveness of lymphocytes
1960	Porter and Edelman elucidate the structure of an antibody
1966–7	Cloman, Davies and Mitchison describe co-operation between B- and T-lymphocytes
1969	International Union of Immunological Societies founded. *Immunological Reviews* begins publication
1971	First International Congress of Immunology in Washington
1971	Gershan reports suppression by T-lymphocytes
1974	Jerne describes the network theory of immuno-regulation
1975	Kohler and Milstein fuse mouse lymphocytes and myeloma cells to generate monoclonal antibody
1977	Smallpox eradicated
1980	Ollsson and Kaplan produce human hybridomas
1984	Davis and Hedrick resolve nature of T-lymphocyte antigen receptor

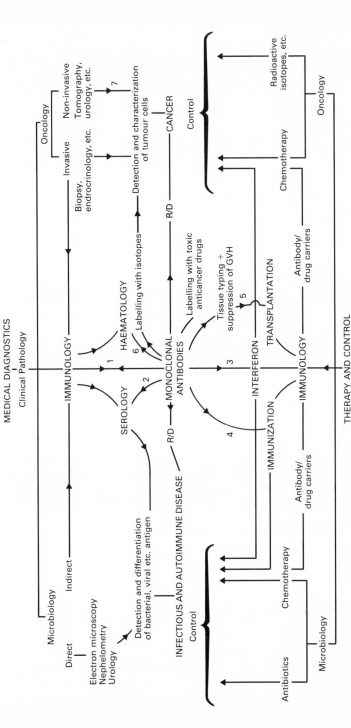

Figure 1.1   Applications of monoclonal antibodies in immunology and related disciplines.
Key: 1, Analysis of the workings of the immune system. 2, Improvement of serological tests and also purification of antigens for antibody detection: ELISA, fluorescent antibody test, radioimmunoassay, etc. 3, Purification of interferon. 4, Purification of antigens for vaccine production and possible use in passive immunization, e.g. for rabies. 5, Therapeutic application in transplant rejection (graft versus host). 6, Blood grouping improved. 7, Improvement of computer-aided tomography

11. Transplantation: covers immunological tolerance, prevention of graft rejection and tissue typing.

The above presents only one classification scheme; there may be many others, both now and in the future as sub-areas develop and change.

1.3 RELATIONSHIPS WITH OTHER DISCIPLINES

Immunology evolved out of microbiology, chiefly bacteriology, nearly a century ago; and the two have developed symbiotically ever since with a great deal of the earlier immunological research being carried out in departments or institutes of microbiology. Microbiology itself emerged only a little earlier than immunology, when the causes of pathological damage in some diseases were seen to be micro-organisms. Attempts to vaccinate against infectious diseases subsequently led to the origin of immunology.

A close relationship has always existed between immunology (chiefly the study of the white blood cell or leukocyte) and haematology (the study of the red blood cell or erythrocyte). While functionally the two cell types are very different, they circulate intimately together in the arteries and veins of the body. The major blood groups, A, B and O, were distinguished by immunological techniques in 1900. At the turn of the century immunology turned to chemistry and biochemistry to help explain the antibody–antigen combination; so began the age of immunochemistry. Pharmacology, earlier this century, set about the task of finding drugs to counteract histamine release by certain white blood cells. In the 1950s, and thereafter, immunology began to interact with disciplines like genetics and cell and molecular biology to help elucidate questions posed at the molecular, cellular and genetic level of the immunologically responsive cells. In the late 1960s and 1970s the great increase in knowledge of tumour development and treatment owed much to immunological techniques.

The central role immunology has in all these biological sciences, and the cross-fertilization that has resulted, has produced many hybrid disciplines such as immunochemistry, immunopathology, immunopharmacology, immunogenetics and many others. It is likely that this process will continue — immunotoxicology, photoimmunology and reproductive immunology are all developing fields of interest.

Figure 1.2 illustrates the development of immunology.

1.4 THE PROFESSION

Today immunologists are active in all areas of the biological and medical sciences, yet less than 30 years ago few immunologists would have been found outside the clinical laboratory in hospitals.

In 1974 Dent and Caldwell published a survey in *The Biologist* in which they examined the distribution of posts for biologists, including immunologists, as advertised in *Nature* and *New Scientist*. As a comparison the present authors decided to repeat the exercise but this time looking only at posts for immunologists, or jobs where immunology was the major component of the work. Strictly speaking the results we obtained are not directly comparable as Dent and

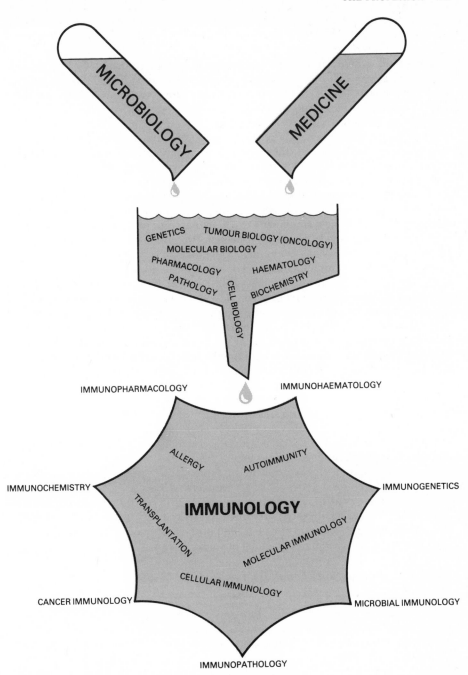

Figure 1.2   Development of immunology

Caldwell did not identify jobs in the private research institutes. Also it is possible that they used different criteria from us to identify the immunology posts. None the less the exercise may prove interesting.

The results are shown in *Table 1.2*. The most striking statistic to emerge from the comparison is that the total number of posts advertised in 1983 had risen by some 50% since 1973. Secondly, whereas in 1973 most posts advertised were for jobs in the government and hospital laboratories, in 1983 most posts were in universities, and a big rise was also seen in the private sector.

These figures do not bear any relationship to the numbers of staff employed by these different organizations, they merely provide an indication of which bodies could actually afford to employ more staff in those particular years. General and wide-ranging cuts in expenditure in the UK's public sector (which includes both government and hospitals) in the 1980s will have accounted for the fall in posts advertised by these bodies in 1983, although the numbers employed are still large. Probably the most significant rise is that seen in industry, where the biotechnology boom, which embraces aspects of immunology such as hybridoma technology, shows few signs of abating. The universities too are growth areas — many of them with commercial links and outlets for their discoveries.

On the face of it then, immunology would appear to offer great prospects for the young biologist at the start of his or her career. However, examination of the details of the advertisements for immunologists in 1983 reveals that the path is far from an easy one. Of the 218 posts, nearly 70% of them specified a PhD as the minimum qualification, with postdoctoral experience being essential for at least half of the posts; 24% demanded an honours degree; and the rest either did not specify, or requested an HNC (a British technical qualification).

It should be noted that advertisements for junior technical posts may not always appear in *Nature* and *New Scientist;* they are more likely to appear in the local or national newspapers such as the *Guardian* or *Daily Telegraph*. None the less entry to the research laboratory requires the achievement of very high qualifications. This 'academic inflation' is characteristic of many other areas of the biomedical sciences, for example virology.

Closer examination of the 1983 immunology posts reveals perhaps a more alarming feature; just under half are university-based short-tenured posts, ranging from one year to a maximum of three years. With the cuts in financial support for the universities and colleges experienced in Europe and the USA, fellows and research assistants in such temporary posts can no longer expect to become part of the permanent teaching or research staff.

Table 1.2   Distribution of immunology posts 1973–83

	Total no. of posts	Percentage of posts advertised				
		Government*	Institutes	Hospitals	Universities	Industry
1973	138	40	No figures available	45	10	5
1983	218	15	10	15	40	20

*Includes Research Councils

The job titles of the permanent posts in our sample included the following: lecturers, professors, research biochemists, basic-grade biochemists and micro-biologists, junior and senior scientists, research managers, technicians, research officers, laboratory chiefs, immunoparasitologists and, of course, but not very frequently, immunologists.

Such is the diversity of immunology.

2 Organizations as information sources

2.1 INTRODUCTION

This chapter and the next provide a comprehensive review of the various professional, academic, research and government agencies that together, admittedly sometimes unwittingly, provide for the well-being and development of immunology.

The commercial firms that operate within the field are also dealt with, but the treatment is necessarily less comprehensive as there are many more of them, and only a few make a meaningful contribution to the subject at large.

There are no authoritative figures available of the number of immunological organizations, but there are certainly over one thousand. A myriad of interlinking organizations service the field; some provide funds for research, others conduct the research themselves; some provide reference facilities, while others actively disseminate information; some provide administrative support to run conferences, short courses, etc., others are policy-making or standard-setting bodies; finally there are those that are concerned with education and training. However most provide a unique and particular blend of services, and all can provide useful information.

In the same way that a journal or book is a source of information so too is an organization. An approach to an organization, whether by letter, phone or personal visit, is often likely to yield information of a higher quality more quickly and easily than the conventional literature search. Furthermore, the information obtained is likely to be more current and the act of obtaining it far less onerous. Not surprisingly this particular method of obtaining information is exceedingly popular, particularly with practitioners whose time is at a premium, many of whom have built up, over a period of time, a network of contacts to refer to for particular kinds of information.

Many organizations also act as information clearing houses, directing the user either to alternative or to additional sources of information, a particularly useful facility because, in the initial stages of the information search, most people's conceptions of what they need are vague (it is not easy to decide what is needed until you are aware of what is available). Many organizations, of course, also publish considerable amounts of information.

2.2 FINDING OUT ABOUT ORGANIZATIONS

(*see* bibliography entries 1–31)

There is unfortunately no one source of information on immunological organizations; instead we have to turn to the directories of science, medicine, biology and biotechnology, and there are many, many, of these.

Directories of organizations funding or conducting research, and research-in-progress lists

The value of such directories and lists is considerable in such a fast and broadly moving field, where few can afford to wait the many months it takes for reports of new developments to appear in the scientific press. Through these tools it is possible to identify individual centres of excellence, and major research studies, and by tuning into the informal information exchange network obtain early intelligence of important developments. It is also likely, in such a young field, that a lot of information will not yet have been written up or published.

Research is, by definition, the creation of new knowledge, knowledge which may have the most important repercussions, and as a consequence information which is highly desirable. This is particularly so in immunology, where prevailing ideas and methods are so transitory. The main problem in chasing immunological research is not a lack of published sources about ongoing research; the problems are incomplete or out-of-date registers, the mass of material to be worked through, the difficulty of physical access to reference sources (particularly those covering other countries) and the lack of co-operation between research workers.

For a global view of immunological research organizations' activities there is the *Medical research index*, which is a world guide to industrial enterprises, hospitals, research laboratories, universities and societies which conduct, promote or encourage research in medicine and related subjects. The work is arranged by country. Differences between the 130 countries covered are marked, with the US obtaining by far the largest entry (168 pages); the UK's entry is 83 pages in length. The index is rudimentary, organizations being indexed by subject words in their title (or translated title). Thus the immunology department of St Jude's Children's Research Hospital is not indexed under immunology (where incidentally 31 organizations may be found). Entries are fairly detailed, though there are variations between entries. The entry for the Österreichische Gesellschaft für Allergologie und Immunologie states, for instance, under scope of activities, 'tumour immunology with special emphasis on immunological aspects of lympho-proliferative diseases'.

A new edition of the work, entitled *Medical research centres*, has been announced for early 1984. It is claimed to cover over 3000 organizations, but most importantly, it is to have an extensive subject index listing such topics as immunization, immunoassay and immunology. The interval between editions is obviously too long for effective intelligence of research activity in the field. The price is very high; currently £175.

Agricultural research centres, a reference tool from the same publishers (Longman), provides a very similar service for agriculture and should be used in conjunction with the above if funds allow (it costs £148).

As expensive ($235 the set), but covering a wider subject area, is *International research centers directory*, published by Gale.

Somewhat narrower in scope, but still providing a multinational view of immunological research, is *European research centres*, the successor to *European research index* and *East European research index*. It is a directory of organizations in science, technology, agriculture and medicine arranged by country — 31 countries in all, including Albania, Cyprus and Iceland. Immunology is listed in the index, which gives a large number of entries, subdivided by country; for example there are 11 Belgian entries and 54 for France. Generally, societies sponsoring research are not given, just bodies active in research. For the UK, most of the immunological research centres are academic, Charing Cross Hospital Medical School's Experimental Pathology Department and Chelsea College's Physiology Department being typical examples. In theory each entry includes: title and address of organization, affiliation, name of research director and senior staff, numbers of graduate research staff, annual expenditure, activities and major projects, contract work and publications. In practice some of the entries are very sparse indeed. The level of detail provided is demonstrated by the entry for the International Immunology Training and Research Centre in Amsterdam, where the section on research activities states rather simply: 'immunology of schistosomiasis, tumour-immunology'. Published irregularly, *European research centres* can never hope accurately to map the rapidly changing face of immunology research in Europe; it does however provide a useful sketch. Perhaps the main criticism of this two-volume work is its price, which at £170 seems exorbitant and well out of the reach of most specialist libraries.

For keeping in touch with immunological research in the USA and Canada, *Research Centers Directory*, and its updating service *New Research Centers*, are indispensable tools. The *Directory* is published every three years and is essentially a guide to research in universities and independent non-profit-making organizations. These organizations are arranged in broad subject categories with the one headed 'Life Sciences' being of most interest, although somewhat daunting with its 1200 or so entries, subdivided by state. It is possible to identify immunology research centres either by browsing through this section, or far better, by using the subject index, where over 100 organizations are listed (unfortunately the index only supplies their location number, so a long search is in prospect). Many of them are of peripheral interest, but as there is no way of telling this from the index it is necessary to scan them all.

Each centre is described in about 12–15 lines, giving, among other things, names of those involved, address, principal activities, and publications. The entry for the Armana Hammar Center for Cancer Biology gives a detailed eight-line statement on its research activities, albeit in a rather bland tone (i.e. 'areas of research include virology, immunology, . . .'). The entry for the Center for Interdisciplinary Research in Immunological Diseases at UCLA usefully provides a note that the Center maintains a library on asthma, allergy and immunology. The basic directory is updated by the thrice-yearly *New Research Centers*, and while it provides no subject index, the number of entries is probably small enough to allow browsing, certainly if the search is restricted to the Life Sciences section; though there are dangers in such an approach in such an interdisciplinary field. Around a dozen immunological organizations are featured in each issue — a sign of the rising fortunes of the field, and a demonstration of the need for currency in this field.

A competitor to the above is the rather more specialized *Research Programs in the Medical Sciences (RPMS)*, which lists 1600 manufacturing and industrial service concerns, academic and non-profit-making organizations, and 5000 departments doing research. It is arranged alphabetically by name of the organization; there is an accompanying research subject index. Published biennially, *RPMS* is not as current as *Research Centers Directory*.

A less conventional approach to listing US research in progress is offered by the Smithsonian Science Information Exchange (SSIE) computer database, which can be accessed via DIALOG (*SSIE Current Research*). This database now contains summaries of research initiated or completed during the period 1978–82. Project descriptions have been obtained from 1300 organizations, mainly government agencies, but academic and private organizations also contributed. The database contains almost half a million citations to research projects, and biological and medical sciences are covered in some depth. There are 4000 references to immunological research projects. SSIE is now a closed file; however, updated information on Federally funded research only may be obtained from another DIALOG database, *Federal Research in Progress*. This file covers such important research funders as the National Institutes of Health and the Department of Agriculture. Of the 70 000 or so mainly scientific projects listed, 2500 are immunological in nature. Semi-annual re-loads keep the file fairly current.

Two other useful US research guides should also be mentioned. These are the *National biomedical research directory* and the *Research Awards Index*, both produced by the US National Institutes of Health.

Within the UK, fair coverage of research in progress is provided by three publications: *Research in British Universities, Polytechnics and Colleges*, which provides a listing of academic research, *Industrial research in the United Kingdom*, which provides a comprehensive picture of research in industrial firms, public corporations, research organizations, government departments and academic bodies; and the *Medical research directory*, another largely academic publication.

The coverage of the widely available *Research in British Universities, Polytechnics and Colleges*, an annual directory published by the British Library, is self-explanatory. Volume 2, *Biological Sciences*, is of prime interest to immunologists. Research projects are listed under their respective host institutions, and these are in turn grouped according to their subject areas. Unfortunately immunology does not have its own section; projects are scattered throughout the volume, chiefly under 'Medical and biomedical science', but also under 'Medicine', 'Microbiology' and 'Zoology'. To locate all these the user needs the subject index; however, the immune/immunology keywords and their variants cover nearly three pages. Most of the projects listed started in 1981/82 and were due to finish 1983/84. Only the bare minimum of information is provided; this directory is really to be used as a signposting service.

Industrial research in the United Kingdom: a guide to organizations and programmes is now in its tenth edition (1983) and is a long-running reference work. The latest volume, the publishers say, places a new emphasis on biotechnology. Thirty-nine immunological organizations can be traced through the index (the main body of the work being organized, unhelpfully, by type of organization — i.e. industrial firms, universities and polytechnics) but despite its title and the alleged coverage of over a thousand industrial, official, and other laboratories, none is an industrial firm. The kinds of organization covered in immunology can be gauged from the following list: the Blond McIndie Centre for Medical Research, Queen Victoria Hospital, East Grinstead; the South Wales Cancer Research Council; the Marine Biological Station at Millport, Strathclyde; and St Mary's Hospital Medical School, University of London. The standard directorial data are supplied for the entries, but also given is annual research expenditure, and a 4–12 line activities statement. While the index does allow for specific searching (i.e. drugs, anti-cancer), retrieval on monoclonal antibodies or hybridoma technology is not possible. Research centres or departments with a research expenditure of less than £30,000 p.a. are omitted.

New to the field is *The medical research directory*, which appeared for the first time in 1983. It is published by John Wiley and its scope is British. Abstracts of over 25,000 research projects currently being undertaken in hospitals, National Health Service organizations, universities and medical schools, and private research establishments, are provided. The work is in fact based upon — and owes much to — *Research in British Universities, Polytechnics and Colleges (RBUPC)* but augments this with information from the Medical Research Council, other research councils, and charitable trusts. Projects are listed by broad subject heading, one of which is immunology, where approximately 400 projects can be located, these being listed by the name of the institution in which the research is conducted. Included in the immunology entry is the work of the National Institute for Medical Research, the MRC Immunology Team at Guy's Hospital and the Agricultural Research Council. As immunology is such a multi-disci-plinary topic and the editors place all work of a department together (despite subject differences), consultation of the index is a must if a comprehensive picture is to be obtained. A brief glance at the index (which is quite specific, giving such entries as immune complex and immune response) shows immunological research listed in the haematology, dermatology, biochemistry, cancer, microbiology and epidemiology subject sections. A problem with these irregular print productions is that some of the research being read about in 1984 will in fact have been completed in 1981/1982. Whether the *Directory* is worth three times the price being asked for *RBUPC* only time will tell.

Not to be ignored are the specialist research grant and award lists of the principal funding organizations such as the Department of Health and Social Security, which publishes the *DHSS Handbook of Research and Development*, and the Medical Research Council, which publishes the *Medical Research Council Handbook*. These lists are valuable as they are so complete.

Guides to biotechnology companies

A recent issue of *Immunology Today* (**5** (3), 1984, 58–9) contained a critical review of a selection of guides devoted to the commercial and academic aspects of bio-technology; all were published in 1983 or 1984. They included: *The new biotech-nology marketplace: the Telegen directory of Japanese biotechnology* (1983); *The Telegen directory of US biotechnology* (1983); *The guide to corporate sponsored university research in biotechnology* (1983); McGraw-Hill's *Biotechnology NEWSWATCH* (1983); *Genetic engineering and biotechnology yearbook 1983* (1983); and *Commercial biotechnology: an international analysis* (1984).

Registers of foundations and grant-giving bodies

Tracing organizations providing grants for research and study in immunology is made relatively straightforward thanks to four on-line databases: *Foundation Directory*, *Foundation Grants Index*, *Grants* and *National Foundations*; all four are available on DIALOG.

Foundation Directory (FD) states which US organizations will provide funds for research. It lists 3500 foundations which have assets of $1 million or more, or which make grants of $100 000 or more annually. They are all non-governmen-tal, non-profit-making, tax-deductable charitable organizations. A lengthy purpose and activities section accompanies each record, and usefully gives the funds available, and guidelines for applications. The database is updated twice yearly. *Foundation Grants Index* (*FGI*) is a companion file which lists projects that have been carried out under Foundation grants, from 400 of the major foundations covered by the former database. It gives a better idea of the likelihood that any particular organization will provide funds because it is based upon its previous funding record. The best way to use the two databases is to look up research projects on immunology on *FGI* and then turn to *FD* for full application details. *FGI* in fact currently (April 1984) lists 200 immunology research grants.

It is also possible to search for grants awarded in much more specific areas, such as immunoresponse (1 given) and immunoregulation (2). The file can be searched back to 1973, and updating is carried out bimonthly (grants are listed approximately three months after they have been awarded). It is possible to search for grants awarded to foreign organizations, and for studying certain population groups such as women, children and the aged.

Grants can be used to extend the scope of *Foundation Directory* for it covers government, commercial organizations and associations, as well as foundations; it is also rather more international in scope, with around one-fifth of the organizations being non-American. Information includes money availability, limitations, geographical restrictions, form of proposal, and a fairly detailed abstract covering scope of activities, etc. Around 2000 organizations are listed on this monthly updated file, over 30 of which offer grants in the broad field of immunology, and as many as 5 provide funds for immunotherapy.

National Foundations provides a very similar service to *Foundation Directory* but lists US organizations — many of them local — regardless of their assets, adding another 18 000 entries to *Foundation Directory*'s total.

Two other publications of interest (only available in print) are the *Directory of grant-making trusts*, mentioned largely for its coverage of the UK and Commonwealth, and *The Grants Register*, which lists bodies awarding grants for educational courses or programmes. The *Directory of grant-making trusts* is a guide to sources of charitable funds, and gives details of over 2300 bodies, with a total income of nearly £400 million. A classified subject index does not provide the necessary detail to locate directly those trusts funding immunological research, and instead one has to browse through such entries as: sciences, agriculture; sciences, biochemistry; and medicine and health, arthritis. *The Grants Register* does in fact enable a direct approach via its index, through such terms as immunology (3 bodies given), biotechnology (1) and allergy (2). Of course many organizations offering medical grants will in fact sponsor immunological research. The *Register* is intended for students at, or above, graduate level, and for all who require further professional or advanced vocational training. Scholarships, exchange opportunities, competitions and vocational awards are all listed. The scope of this work is international.

The many societies and professional organizations that exist in the field can be traced in a variety of publications: *Encyclopedia of associations* (American), *Trade associations and professional bodies of the United Kingdom*, *Directory of British Associations*, *Directory of European scientific organizations*, *World guide to scientific associations* and *World of learning*. They all have subject indexes which enable medical, biological, and sometimes immunological, societies to be identified. The *Encyclopedia of associations* is the largest and most detailed of them all, covering 15 000 organizations, and providing an abstract of the scope, purpose and major activities of each organization; it is available in hard copy and machine-readable form (via DIALOG). It lists 39 immunological organizations but most are only of peripheral interest. The *Encyclopedia of medical organizations and agencies* lists some 10 000 organizations; medical schools, foundations and research centres are included. They are all arranged by broad subject (e.g. biomedical engineering).

For tracing international organizations in immunology, the *Yearbook of International Organizations* is particularly useful (a detailed subject index provides access to purely immunological organizations) and authoritative (it is published by the Union of International Associations).

Directories of libraries and information services

Two directories offer comprehensive coverage of US immunological information resources: the *Directory of Health Science Libraries in the United States*, which arranges its data geographically, and *Medical and Health Information Directory*, which offers an alternative form of organization by activity (i.e. publishing). The *Directory of Health Science Libraries in the United States* lists 2755 sources, including on-line database services, while the *Medical and Health Information Directory*, which interprets information sources rather more broadly, boasts a coverage of 16 000 medical libraries, information centres, research centres, information systems, publishers, medical schools, etc. Both are irregularly published, and both were published last in 1983.

The *Aslib directory of information sources in the United Kingdom*: vol. 1, *Science, technology and commerce* is the definitive guide to British information sources (the term is used very broadly). The index must be used to locate immunological libraries and information services; 18 are listed. Most are general libraries that have specialist collections in immunology, such as Glasgow University Library, Cambridge University Pathology Library and Paddington College Library. However, the British Society for Immunology, the British Society for Allergy and Clinical Immunology (a society in name only) and the Wellcome Research Laboratories are also given.

For an international view of immunological information resources *World guide to special libraries* is probably most useful. The work is arranged by broad subject; the section for Medicine and Life Science lists 4500 libraries from well over a hundred countries. A simple subject index provides for more specific subject requirements.

3 Organizations in immunology

3.1 INTRODUCTION

As in many other areas of science, immunological research is dominated by workers from the USA. While it is arguable that the Americans are not always as innovative as the Europeans — most of the major immunological breakthroughs, such as monoclonal antibody production, have been made in the UK and Europe — they do have a remarkable talent for utilizing ideas.

An examination of the 1982 volumes of *Journal of Immunology* and *Immunology* reveals that about half of all the papers were published by American authors (*see Figure 3.1*). Of these, by far the majority had been written by researchers from universities and medical schools. The government and independent research institutes provided roughly equal numbers of papers amounting to just under a third of the US total. A small but increasingly significant number came from the commercial sector.

The next major contributors were the British, supplying about 10% of all papers. The British universities and medical schools contributed over a half of these, with the government laboratories providing somewhat less than half. Independent institutes and private companies accounted for the remainder.

The Japanese were responsible for over 6% of all papers, the universities publishing the lion's share and the government providing the rest. The reverse is true in France, which accounts for 5.5% of all papers, where government employment is the most prolific source of authors. The majority of papers by West German authors, who were responsible for 5% of all papers published, came from the universities, with the remainder coming from the autonomous research institutes. A similar situation exists in Canada (total contribution 4.5%) with the universities being the dominant body. In Switzerland (3%) there was a fairly even mix between universities, research institutes, government and commercial companies. Australian and Swedish research (2.5%) appears evenly divided between universities and government; and papers issued from the Netherlands are virtually all from university researchers.

3.2 INTERNATIONAL ORGANIZATIONS

International Union of Immunological Societies (IUIS)

The IUIS was officially founded in 1969 by representatives of 10 national

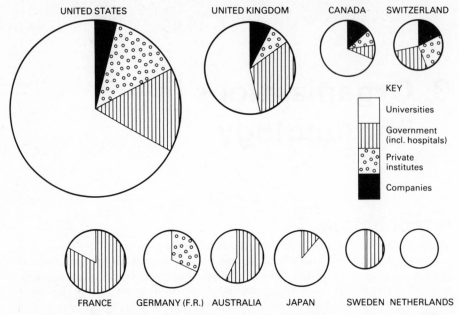

*Figure 3.1   Workplace of authors of immunological papers. Data are com-
piled from the 1982 volumes of* Journal of Immunology *and* Immunology.
The areas of the circles are proportional to the numbers of papers

societies: the American Association of Immunologists, the British Society for
Immunology, the Canadian Society for Immunology, the Dutch Society for
Immunology, the Gesellschaft für Immunologie (FRG), the Israel Immunologi-
cal Society, the Polish Society of Immunology, the Scandinavian Society for
Immunology, the Société Française d'Immunologie and the Yugoslav
Immunological Society. The Australian Society for Immunology and the Swiss
Society of Allergy, although not represented at the inauguration, were also
declared to be founding members.

Thirty-three national societies are presently full members of IUIS, the most
recent members being those societies from the People's Republic of China and
Taiwan — a move designed to circumvent political barriers to scientific exchange
amongst immunologists (*see* directory entries 543–576). In addition, a number of
national societies have observer status pending their formal acceptance by IUIS;
these include the societies of Czechoslovakia, Iran, Singapore and the Soviet
Union.

In 1976 IUIS was accepted as a member of the International Council of
Scientific Unions (ICSU). Curiously this honour has been denied the longer-
established International Union of Microbiological Societies (IUMS). Membership of the ICSU does confer influence (i.e. numbers of votes) on such important
bodies as the Royal Society, which advises the British government on scientific
matters.

The aims of the IUIS are:

1. To organize international co-operation in immunology and to promote communication between the various branches of immunology and allied subjects.
2. To encourage within each country co-operation between the societies that represent the interests of immunology.
2. To contribute to the advancement of immunology in all its aspects.

Organization

The IUIS is governed by 16 members who constitute the Council. The Council is divided into seven committees:

1. The Education Committee promotes and organizes courses in developing countries, and supports permanent centres for international immunology training, in collaboration with international agencies such as the ICSU, Unesco and the WHO.

2. The Nomenclature Committee is concerned with standardizing immunological terminology — an extremely important exercise in such a rapidly developing field. The committee comprises 10 subcommittees which deal with specific areas such as hybridomas, lymphokines, complement and thymic hormones. Some of the subcommittees are jointly organized by the IUIS and other international organizations like the Reticulo-endothelial Society (RES) and the WHO.

3. The Standardization Committee comprises IUIS members, and liaison members of other national and international societies such as the International Association of Biological Standardization (IABS), the European Committee for Clinical Laboratory Standards (ECCLS), the National Committee for Clinical Laboratory Standards (NCCLS) and the National Institute for Biological Standardization and Control (NIBSC). It in turn possesses 16 subcommittees covering areas such as histocompatibility, tumour markers and human immunoglobulins. The many activities of the Standardization Committee include: fostering the development of immunological research standards and arranging for their preparation; examination, storage and distribution; writing specifications for selected immunological reagents; and disseminating information to promote acceptance and establishment of immunological research standards.

The work of the Standardization Committee is intimately bound up with that of the WHO. Indeed a joint IUIS/WHO programme, initiated in 1973, establishes priorities and practical methods, at regular meetings of the two bodies, as to the best ways to meet the most urgent needs.

4. The Symposium Committee, as its name suggests, organizes the annual symposia and selects the topics and venues. In general the meetings last 4–5 days, and, curiously, the proceedings are never published.

5. The Clinical Immunology Committee works together with the national immunological societies and the WHO Immunology Unit in establishing and organizing departments and centres for clinical immunology. It provides training opportunities in this area, as well as evaluating and standardizing immunological tests. The work of the Committee is guided by the WHO Technical Report on clinical immunology (No. 496, 1972) which outlines the basis for the application of immunology for the benefit of patients.

6. The Veterinary Immunology Committee facilitates the exchange of information among veterinary immunologists, is responsible for the improvement of standards of education for veterinary students in immunology, and transfers information on immunological problems in domestic animals, to non-veterinary immunologists. The committee consists of 18 members equally representing Europe, North America and the rest of the world.

7. Finally **the Publication Committee,** which is the most recently established committee, deals with the future publication policy of the IUIS.

Meetings

A great many meetings take place under the auspices of the IUIS, sometimes with and sometimes without assistance from other bodies, such as the WHO. But undoubtedly the most important meeting is the International Congress of Immunology. The 1st International Congress was held in Washington, D.C., in 1971 and represented a milestone in the emergence of immunology as an independent scientific discipline. A surprisingly high number of immunologists participated (3400), representing 45 countries. Since then there have been Congresses every three years: Brighton 1974; Sydney 1977; Paris 1980; and Kyoto 1983. Future Congresses are to be held in Toronto in 1986 and Berlin in 1989. The proceedings have all been published (*see* section 4.4).

The Symposium Committee also holds annual meetings on individual topics which are chiefly aimed at giving young immunologists an opportunity to participate at international discussion meetings which are generally limited to between 100 and 200 people. The 14th conference was held in the Tyrol in 1984. The proceedings of these meetings are never published.

Relationships with other bodies

The IUIS collaborates with numerous national and international organizations, a number of which have already been mentioned: WHO, ICSU, Unesco, RES, IABS, ECCLS, NCCLS and the NIBSC.

The IUIS is also an associate member of the Council for International Organizations of Medical Sciences (CIOMS). There are also relationships with the European Molecular Biology Organization (EMBO), the International Reticulo-endothelial Society and the International College of Allergologists.

Within the framework of the IUIS, the European societies of immunology have established a European Federation, which is entitled to hold its own meetings.

In 1982 the International Society for Immunopharmacology was admitted as an Affiliated Commission of the IUIS because this would 'promote an orderly interaction with an interdisciplinary group and a link between immunology and pharmacology'.

Hybridoma and monoclonal antibody data bank

A data bank has been created by the IUIS which collects, codes, stores and distributes information on all lines and hybridomas making monoclonal or immunological active factors.

Table 3.1. ‾ *Leading national societies of immunology affiliated to the IUIS*

Country	IUIS member since	Membership (1981)
USA	1969	3045
Japan	1970	2400
UK	1969	2053
Netherlands	1969	790
Scandinavia	1969	727
Federal Republic of Germany	1969	663
France	1969	550
Poland	1969	448
Italy	1971	415
Australia	1969	375
Canada	1969	360
Hungary	1973	350

World Health Organization (WHO)

The WHO, a specialized agency of the United Nations founded in 1947, plays an extremely active role in immunology: it researches, trains, provides funds, organizes meetings, publishes and advises.

The work of the WHO is largely conducted through a number of advisory groups and committees. *Figure 3.2* illustrates the part of the structure of the WHO which is of special interest to immunology. To each division within an advisory group a number of Expert Advisory Panels report, the main one concerning immunology being the Immunology Unit. Of some significance also are the Bacterial Diseases, Virus Diseases and the Biological Standardization Units.

Much of the immunological work with which the WHO is involved is of an applied nature in the area of human and animal disease: understanding the immunological reaction in bacterial, viral and parasitic diseases; standardization and production of reagents and techniques; production of better vaccines such as that against dengue haemorrhagic fever; carrying out serological surveys; and assessing the socio-economic importance of allergic reactions in the developing countries.

More recently work has centred on the immunological diseases such as the autoimmune diseases and rheumatoid arthritis.

The WHO Immunology Research and Training Centres, now forming a world-wide network, are carrying out much of this research in close co-operation with local institutions. These centres train scientists, particularly from the developing countries, on an individual basis or through organized courses. Such courses have taken place in Nairobi, São Paulo, Lausanne, New Delhi and Asyut (Egypt).

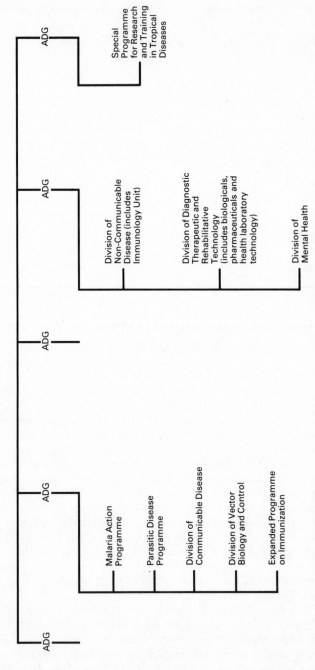

DIRECTOR GENERAL

ADG

ADG

ADG

ADG

ADG

Malaria Action Programme

Parasitic Disease Programme

Division of Communicable Disease

Division of Vector Biology and Control

Expanded Programme on Immunization

Division of Non-Communicable Disease (includes Immunology Unit)

Division of Diagnostic Therapeutic and Rehabilitative Technology (includes biologicals, pharmaceuticals and health laboratory technology)

Division of Mental Health

Special Programme for Research and Training in Tropical Diseases

Figure 3.2   The WHO's Headquarter Secretariat showing its immunology and immunology-related activities

The WHO has also provided a comprehensive reference service based upon existing national laboratories. As well as the WHO Collaborating Centres, as they are known, covering specific diseases such as influenza, leprosy and malaria, there are a total of 35 concerned with immunology alone, studying complement deficiency, immunoglobulins, leukocyte antigens, and many other areas. (The names and addresses of these laboratories are listed as directory entries 590–617).

Relationship with other bodies

A close relationship exists between the IUIS and the WHO. Official relations started in 1972. The Immunology Unit of the WHO has observer status on the Council, and representatives on the Standardization and Clinical Immunology Committees, of the IUIS. Many meetings are jointly supported by the two bodies.

Publications

The major publications for disseminating information on its activities are: *Bulletin of the World Health Organzation*, a scholarly journal which regularly reports on the status of infectious and non-infectious diseases worldwide (in 1981, **51,** pp. 717–28, it reported on a meeting conducted with the IUIS on a collaborative review of some of the most frequently used tests in clinical immunology); the *WHO Chronicle*, a monthly newsletter containing general information on the principal activities of the WHO including news of conferences, meetings, and funding; and *The Work of the WHO*, which is the official biennial record of its activities.

Much of the WHO's research and missives on standards and techniques are contained in two report series: the *Monograph Series* (2–3 are published a year); and the *Technical Report Series* (some 100 reports might be issued every year). The *Technical Report Series* also includes the official reports of the work of the various Expert Committees such as that for Biological Standardization; one of the most recent of these is the 33rd Report which is contained in Technical Report Series 687 (1983).

European Committee for Clinical Laboratory Standards

The formation of the European Committee for Clinical Laboratory Standards (ECCLS), inspired largely by the US National Committee for Clinical Laboratory Standards (NCCLS), a much older body with which it collaborates extensively, occurred in 1979. The activities of the ECCLS are essentially concerned with the quality of clinical laboratory results. Their purpose is to inform scientists in the health agencies, in industry and in clinical laboratories about progress in clinical laboratory standards. Membership, now at 161, is open to professional societies, health authorities, industrial organizations and individuals.

The ECCLS organizes meetings, seminars and international conferences on clinical laboratory standards and organization. It publishes the quarterly *ECCLS News*, which contains news, reports of meetings and a mini-directory listing the composition of all ECCLS bodies.

International Association of Allergology

The International Association of Allergology (IAA) was founded in 1945 and today represents 39 national societies, including the British Society for Allergy and Clinical Immunology. Its object is to further work in the educational, research, and practical medical aspects of allergic diseases. Like the IUIS it is a member of the CIOMS, other members of which include the International League against Rheumatism and the Collegium Internationale Allergologium.

Meetings are generally organized by the relevant national societies.

Collegium Internationale Allergologicum

The Collegium Internationale Allergologicum is a small, highly exclusive society founded in 1965 for those physicians especially interested in the study of scientific and clinical problems in allergy, and related branches of medicine and immunology. It conducts scientific meetings and symposia, the highlights being the biennial symposia. The 1982 symposium was held in Sorrento. The 12th Symposium was held in New Orleans in 1978, and the proceedings were published as volume 14 of *Monographs in Allergy*, entitled *New approaches to the management of allergic diseases* (1979).

The Collegium is an associate member of the International Association of Allergology.

European Academy of Allergology and Clinical Immunology

The European Academy of Allergology and Clinical Immunology is based in Rome. Its chief purpose appears to be organizing the Annual Congress of the European Academy of Allergology and Clinical Immunology. The 12th Congress was held in Rome in 1983 and co-sponsored by the Italian Society of Allergology and Clinical Immunology, under the auspices of the WHO.

European Molecular Biology Organization

Financed jointly by the major European countries with its headquarters in Heidelberg, the European Molecular Biology Organization (EMBO) promotes collaboration in the field of molecular biology and awards fellowships for training and research in the same. Its most visible activities are the organizing of workshops and courses; there may be as many as 20 of each every year. In 1983 it held workshops entitled 'Towards new vaccines' and 'Histocompatibility systems', and practical courses entitled 'Antigen specific T-cell lines' and 'Antibodies in cell biology'. The workshops and conferences are held mainly in West Germany, England, Switzerland and the Netherlands.

EMBO also publishes a monthly journal, *The EMBO Journal*, which carries a significant amount of immunological research.

European Federation of Immunological Societies

Within the framework of the IUIS, the European societies of immunology decided to establish a European Federation of Immunological Societies (EFIS). Its first meeting was in Strasbourg in 1973. Subsequent meetings have taken place irregularly; the most recent were held in Turkey (1982) and Switzerland (1984).

The objects of EFIS are to promote closer contact and co-operation between immunological societies in Europe, and to facilitate the exchange of scientific information and scientific workers.

EFIS's most notable achievement to date is the publication of the journal *Immunology Letters*, a vehicle for the rapid dissemination of immunological research.

Transplantation Society

The Transplantation Society is open to physicians and others who have made significant contributions to the advancement of knowledge in transplantation biology and medicine. Its purpose is a simple one — to further knowledge in this area. It was founded in 1966 and today has 1400 members, mainly American. The Society presents awards and holds biennial congresses: the 9th International Congress of the Transplantation Society was held in Brighton in 1982; the next is to be held in Minneapolis in 1984. Its two major publications are *Transplantation* (monthly) and *Transplantation Proceedings* (quarterly).

International Association of Biological Standardization

The International Association of Biological Standardization (IABS) founded in 1955, is an independent commission of the International Union of Microbiological Societies, which also has close ties with the WHO's Expert Committee on Biological Standardization. A relationship exists too with the Standardization Committee of the IUIS; indeed their objectives and activities are very similar.

The aims of IABS are to promote the development and use of standardized techniques, and to support the work of the WHO in the study and application of international biological standards, reference preparations and reagents.

Of the meetings which IABS organizes, the biennial international congresses (where problems relating to research, production and control of immunological products are discussed) and the twice-yearly symposia are most relevant to immunologists. The proceedings are published as *Developments in Biological Standardization* but were previously known as *Progress in Immunological Standardization* and the *Symposia Series in Immunobiological Standardization*.

IABS also publishes a quarterly journal entitled *Journal of Biological Standardization*.

International Society of Developmental and Comparative Immunology

The newly founded International Society of Developmental and Comparative Immunology (ISDCI) promotes the growth of interest in developmental and comparative immunology. Up to 1983 it was responsible for organizing two major international conferences respectively held in Aberdeen in 1980 and in Kyoto, Japan in 1983. The proceedings of the 1st Congress are available as *Aspects of Developmental and Comparative Immunology 1; Proceedings of the 1st Congress of Developmental and Comparative Immunology* and were published by Pergamon in 1981. The ISDCI's official journal, also published by Pergamon, is entitled *Developmental and Comparative Immunology*.

3.3 OTHER SOCIETIES

A number of other societies may be of some interest to immunologists. The International Union of Microbiological Societies (IUMS), embracing 49 national microbiological societies, supervises the work of a number of specialist committees and commissions of which the Committee of Microbiological and Immunological Documentation, and the Commission of Biological Standardization (*see* IABS), are perhaps of most interest.

The World Association of Veterinary Microbiologists, Immunologists and Specialists in Infectious Diseases (WAVMI) is concerned with the problems of domestic animals; in fact its meetings are usually held in conjunction with the World Veterinary Congress.

3.4 COMMERCIAL COMPANIES

The majority of companies active in immunology operate on a multi-national basis. The activities of these companies, in immunology, may be classified into five areas. First, they may manufacture reagents and equipment for laboratory use: antisera, enzyme-labelled and radioactive labelled conjugates, plastic-ware for growing cells and carrying out tests. Secondly, they may produce ethical pharmaceuticals such as vaccines and drugs for both human and animal health care. Thirdly, they may provide medical laboratory services through their own clinical laboratories. Fourthly, they may conduct their own research. Finally, they may fund the research of others.

Obviously, there are some companies that are involved in all five roles, such as the Smith Klein Corporation and the Wellcome Foundation, while there are others whose activities are much more limited in scope.

As has already been shown, the commercial companies do make a significant contribution to immunological research and some companies actively encourage publication of their results. Expenditure on research and development does appear to have increased quite considerably over the last 20 years. A survey by the Association of British Pharmaceuticals Industry (ABPI), the trade association representing 150 manufacturers of prescription medicines (many of them British subsidiaries of multinational companies), showed that spending on R & D was £7.5 million in 1960, £20 million in 1970, and £419.3 million in 1982.

But for those companies where secrecy pervades, even where proprietary rights have been gained, it is exceedingly difficult to find out what research is being carried out; the companies' annual reports are the only guide and a rather superficial one at that.

At the forefront of the commercial interest in immunology is the huge Hoffman-La Roche company. Roche Products Ltd, the pharmaceutical subsidiary, is one of the world's leading drug manufacturers, producing many anti-inflammatory or anti-rheumatic drugs. The company's research and development takes place in four major international research centres, located in the UK, Switzerland, the USA and West Germany. At Welwyn Garden City in England, the work covers the development of *in vitro* assays for cellular and humoral immune responses, and evaluation of immuno-active peptides. A major contribution to immunology was the founding of the Basel Institute for Immunology in 1968. This institute is entirely supported by the company but has full academic freedom. Administratively the Institute is responsible to seven directors, four of whom are La Roche employees.

The Wellcome Foundation, which comprises a total of 60 companies located throughout the world, researches, manufactures and sells medical and veterinary pharmaceuticals, biological products and diagnostic reagents. The company is one of the leading manufacturers of interferon and, in collaboration with the AFRC, produces a live virus vaccine which is used against foot-and-mouth disease. Other research activities include development of a new parvovirus vaccine for dogs, and a rabies vaccine for domestic animals.

The Foundation, through a subsidiary, the Wellcome Trust, allocated £24.5 million during 1980–2 to support medical research and medical history. This budget was used to finance projects (15 in clinical immunology and two in basic immunology) carried out at UK medical schools. In addition a number of senior fellowships for clinical scientists wishing to concentrate fully on research were provided: in 1981 three of the nine recipients were investigating immunological aspects of disease.

The Smith Klein Corporation, like Wellcome, is active in a great many areas: pharmaceuticals, medicines, vaccines, instrumentation. It also provides diagnostic services through a network of clinical laboratories in North America, gives support to a range of medical and scientific programmes, and has created foundations for the advancement of knowledge in medical sciences in Europe.

Other companies active in the field include: Celltech (monoclonal antibodies against interferon); Centocor (kit for hepatitis detection using monoclonal antibodies); Eli Lily (T-lymphocyte hybridomas); Hybritech (monoclonal antibodies against hepatitis B); Hoechst (multivalent vaccines with improved pasteurella component); Intervet (two new animal vaccines produced by recombinant DNA technology); ICI (studies on the secretory immune system and immuno-regulation system); May & Baker Limited (anti-arthritic product); Glaxo (parvovirus vaccine and histamine antagonist); Merck, Sharp & Dohme (vaccine against hepatitis B); and Merrel Pharmaceuticals (drug for histamine-mediated allergies).

The supply of immunoglobulins, reagents and equipment to hospital, research and teaching laboratories is a very important function of the commercial sector. *Table 3.2* lists the main suppliers to immunology laboratories in the UK, and gives an indication of the range of products. A more detailed guide may be found in *Nature's Directory of biologicals — 1983 buyers guide* (1983). Another source of information is the 'immunological product review' (**295,** 1982, 5847) and 'monoclonal antibody product review' (**304,** 1983, 5921) contained in the weekly journal *Nature* from time to time (usually annually). *Linscott's Directory of immunological and biological reagents* (1982–83) is a computer compilation of the products listed in the latest available catalogue of over 200 suppliers of mainly immunological products. Finally, a highly specialized (and now rather dated) index of immunological reagents and equipments is contained in *Practical immunology* by Hudson and Hay (2nd edn, 1980).

3.5 NATIONAL ORGANIZATIONS — UK

Government bodies

The UK has a long history of both direct and indirect governmental involvement

Table 3.2. Some UK-based companies supplying immunology laboratories

	Immunoglobulins and sera	Labelled immunoglobulins	Monoclonal antibodies	Enzymes	Immunochemicals	Biochemical compounds	Diagnostic reagents	Cell separation media	Cell cultures and media	Plastics and glassware	Immunological equipment	Laboratory animals
Amersham		✓	✓									
Boehringer	✓			✓								
Dynatech	✓	✓	✓		✓							
Flow							✓		✓	✓	✓	
Gibco	✓								✓	✓	✓	
New England Nuclear		✓	✓		✓							
Medix			✓									
Nordic	✓	✓			✓	✓						
Pharmacia								✓				
Serotec	✓		✓									
Sigma					✓	✓	✓	✓				
Tago	✓	✓										
UCB	✓	✓	✓									
Wellcome	✓				✓		✓					
LKB											✓	
Miles	✓	✓	✓		✓							
MRC												✓

in immunological research. In this section the following organizations are included because of their particular relevance to immunology: the Public Health Laboratory Service (PHLS), which is directly financed through the Department of Health and Social Security; and the Medical Research Council (MRC) and Agricultural and Food Research Council (AFRC), which are both funded by parliamentary grants-in-aid, but are also reliant on finance from other sources.

Public Health Laboratory Service

The Public Health Laboratory Service (PHLS), through a network of laboratories in England and Wales, is responsible for the prevention and control of infectious disease, via the community physicians.

Its three main centres are the Central Public Health Laboratory (CPHL) at Colindale, London; the Centre for Applied Microbiology and Research (CAMR) at Porton Down; and the Communicable Disease Surveillance Centre, also at Colindale. There are also five reference laboratories, 11 regional laboratories and 41 area laboratories throughout Britain which carry out routine diagnosis; some research is carried out, generally of a serological nature (e.g. on legionellas, bacteroides and campylobacteric infections).

Immunological techniques are used in nearly all divisions of the CPHL but particularly in the Division of Microbiological Reagents and Quality Control, the Virus Reference Laboratory and the Division of Enteric Pathogens. Much of this work involves comparing and distinguishing microbial isolates from patients.

At CAMR, the work of the Vaccine Research and Production Laboratory includes development of sub-unit vaccines against CMV, and production of monoclonal antibodies against a number of viruses such as herpes simplex and vaccinia. Monoclonal antibodies against LCM is part of the work of the Special Pathogens Reference Laboratory. Research using serological techniques also takes place in the Pathogenic Microbes Research Laboratory.

Medical Research Council

The Medical Research Council (MRC) is assisted by four research boards: the Cell Biology and Disorders Board; the Neurobiology and Mental Health Board; the Physiological Systems and Disorders Board; and the Tropical Medicine Research Board. MRC expenditure on research into the immune system amounted to £15 million, or about 15% of its entire income, in 1982.

Most of the immunological research carried out by the MRC takes place under the aegis of the Cell Biology and Disorders Board at the MRC's National Institute for Medical Research (NIMR), the Clinical Research Centre, and at the MRC Units at hospitals and universities throughout the UK. Some of their recent projects include:

Monoclonal antibodies to histocompatibility HLA antigens, viral antigens and tumour antigens, and their application in haematology and in immunoassay to provide a means for accurate assessment of biological substances; the use of monoclonal antibodies as drug carriers (NIMR).

Lymphocytes, their cell surface structures, differentiation and functions (MRC, Cellular Immunology Unit, Oxford).

Immune response, relationship between HLA antigen, regulation of, and disease susceptibility (Nuffield Department of Clinical Medicine, Oxford).

Investigation of immunoglobulin genes, their isolation, structural analysis and expression (Laboratory of Molecular Biology, Cambridge).

Interferon, various aspects (MRC Clinical Research Centre in collaboration with the Laboratory of Molecular Biology; the Department of Biological Sciences, Warwick University; and the Department of Biochemistry, Liverpool University).

The MRC Committee on the Development of Vaccination and Immunization Procedures, which comes under the control of the Physiological Systems and Disorders Board, advises on research on vaccination and immunization procedures and also seeks to initiate and co-ordinate laboratory and clinical investigations.

The Tropical Medicines Research Board has initiated a number of projects including the immunological investigation of the pathogenic mycobacteria that cause leprosy, and similar studies on malaria (carried out at the NIMR) and arenaviruses (London School of Hygiene and Tropical Medicine).

The MRC funds the Institute of Cancer Research jointly with the Cancer Research Campaign. It also finances a great deal of research in independent establishments, and directly supervises the work of 60 research teams in universities and medical schools.

Up until late 1983 exclusive rights to MRC discoveries were enjoyed by Celltech, the government-backed UK biotechnology company. Now, however, Celltech's rights are almost entirely restricted to hybridomas.

National Institute for Biological Standards and Control

The National Institute for Biological Standards and Control (NIBSC) is the fairly recent result of a merger between two divisions of the MRC's NIMR: the Divisions of Biological Standards, and Immunological Products Control. It is now a fully independent body under the control of the National Biological Standards Board.

The work of the Institute is mainly applied, and largely concerned with viral vaccines and virulence.

Agricultural and Food Research Council (AFRC)

The AFRC is financed by parliamentary grant-in-aid, the Ministry of Agriculture, Fisheries and Food, the Department of Agriculture and Fisheries for Scotland, and another hundred bodies. The AFRC, in turn, provides research grants for universities and colleges.

As one would expect the work of the AFRC includes research in veterinary immunology. A selection of projects in this field are listed:

Soluble immunosuppressive molecules and tolerance, immunological control of animal growth (the Institute of Animal Physiology, Cambridge, and the Meat Research Institute, Bristol).

Use of recombinant DNA technology for the production of sub-unit vaccines against foot-and-mouth diseases; and monoclonal antibodies against foot-and-mouth disease (the Animal Viral Research Institute, Pirbright). New vaccines against acute pneumonia and calf diarrhoea (the Moredun Institute, Edinburgh). Development of a vaccine against transmissible gastro-enteritis in piglets using molecular biology techniques (Institute for Research on Animal Diseases, Newbury).

Professional associations

British Society of Immunology

Foremost of the bodies that cater for the education and welfare of immunologists in the UK is the British Society of Immunology (BSI). It was founded in 1956 to advance the science of immunology by means of meetings, of which there are usually three a year, and has two journals, *Immunology* and *Clinical and Experimental Immunology*, where members, and others, may publish their work. The 2760 members (1983) are kept informed of the Society's activities by a loose-leaf monthly newsletter and an annual yearbook.

The Society is administered by a committee which, in addition to the 14 BSI members, also consists of representatives of the British Transplantation Society (BTS) and the British Society for Allergy and Clinical Immunology (BSACI). Reciprocal agreements exist whereby representatives of the BSI attend meetings of the BTS and BSACI, ensuring a co-ordinated approach to items of mutual interest. The Society is responsible for the working of the British National Committee for Immunology, which sends a representative to meetings of the IUIS and ICSU.

The BSI organizes a number of meetings every year, generally called 'Spring',

'Summer' and 'Autumn' meetings. In 1983 there were the following: Clinical Immunology Workshop, Birmingham; Avian Immunology, London; IgA Workshop, London; and the Peter Gorer Symposium at the Barbican, London, which was entitled 'Major histocompatibility complex today'. To assist members to attend these and other meetings the society awards bursaries up to a maximum of £50. Funds from the society are also available to local bona fide immunology groups.

The Society holds a register of individuals or departments who are willing to offer research training in immunology leading to a PhD.

Closely allied to the BSI is the Biochemical Immunology Group, which is part of the Biochemical Society. The group jointly organizes meetings and colloquia with the BSI on biochemically related aspects of immunology, for example 'Production and functions of immortalized lymphocytes' (1983) and 'Effector functions of the constant region of immunoglobulin molecules' (1983).

British Society for Allergy and Clinical Immunology

The British Society for Allergy and Clinical Immunology (BSACI), formerly the British Allergy Society, was founded in 1948, and differs from the BSI in that it is concerned more with the allergic and clinical aspects of immunology such as asthma, hypersensitivity, rhinitis, rheumatoid arthritis and eczema. Whereas members of BSI include many science graduates, the dominant force of BSACI is the medical practitioners; total membership is 330 (1980).

The official publication of the society is the bimonthly journal *Clinical Allergy*.

The Society is a member of the International Association of Allergology, is affiliated to the European Academy of Allergy and Clinical Immunology, and has close relationships with the BSI and the British Transplantation Society.

British Transplantation Society

The aims of the British Transplantation Society (BTS) are to advance the study of biological and clinical problems in tissue and organ transplantation, and to consider its social implication. Membership, which totals just over 400, is open to dialysis physicians, transplantation surgeons and immunologists with an interest in transplantation.

The Society holds meetings; the autumn meeting of 1983 included a lecture on the mechanism of tolerance, and a review of current British transplantation procedures.

The Society has close links with the Transplantation Society and the BSI.

Other societies

The Royal Society of Medicine has a section for Clinical Immunology and Allergy. It organizes meetings, usually held at the Royal Postgraduate Medical School. In 1983, 'The structure and function of immunoglobulin genes' and 'Eosinophils in disease' were two topics discussed.

The Royal College of Pathologists also holds meetings of immunological interest: one was 'Developments in bone marrow transplantation' (1984).

The Immunochemistry Club, which was founded by members of the Royal Postgraduate Medical School, held its third meeting there in 1983; discussed were 'Immunocytochemical innovations'.

In Scotland, the Metchnikoff Club, also known as the Edinburgh Immunology

Group, holds meetings and courses, an example being a course on antigen presentation in 1983.

In the north of England, the West Yorkshire Immunology Group holds monthly meetings, usually at the Leeds General Infirmary.

The Interferon Club, based at Warwick University, and still largely informal, aims to keep a register of members interested in interferon, to circulate a newsletter and to organize occasional meetings.

The activities of the Society of General Microbiology may also be of some interest to immunologists.

Universities and colleges

Research

The British universities are an important force in immunological research (*see Table 3.3*). While they are dependent on government finance through the University Grants Committee for their day-to-day running and teaching costs, their research is largely financed by whatever grants they can obtain from outside sources. An examination of 300 projects in immunology listed in *Research in British Universities, Polytechnics and Colleges*, vol. 2 (1983) showed that the major funders of immunological research were the MRC, the Wellcome Trust, the universities themselves and the Arthritis and Rheumatism Council. The results emphasize the importance of the charity organizations in providing money for research.

Table 3.3   Organizations funding immunological research in UK universities

Organization	Percentage of projects funded
Medical Research Council	30
Wellcome Trust	18
Universities	17
Arthritis and Rheumatism Council	10
Health Authorities	5
Leukaemia Research Fund	3
Multiple Sclerosis Society	2
Cancer Research Campaign	2
Muscular Dystrophy Group	2
Action for Crippled Child	2
Cystic Fibrosis Research Trust	1
Asthma Research Council	1
Science and Engineering Research Council	1
Melville Trust	1
Imperial Cancer Research Fund	1
Others	4

Data based on 300 research projects listed in *Research in British Universities, Polytechnics and Colleges*, vol. 2 (1983)

Conversely, financial assistance from the commercial sector is almost non-existent: Gibco and Upjohn are the only companies to figure, even in the 'Others' category of the table.

Immunological research is carried out in many university departments and medical schools in the UK. The interdisciplinary nature of immunology is demonstrated by the fact that research is carried out under many department titles: biochemistry, bacteriology, clinical surgery, allergy and clinical immunology, haematology, neurology, medicine, infectious diseases, zoology, microbiology, immunochemistry, pathology, virology and, of course, immunology.

It would serve no useful purpose if every university department doing immunological research were listed here; instead we have selected those universities we feel are making the most contributions, either in terms of the number of projects in which they are currently engaged, or the number of papers they have recently published in journals such as *Immunology* and the *Journal of Immunology*. Similarly, it is of little value to describe the activities of the departments, as these are numerous and diverse, and constantly changing.

Thus we will provide only a broad outline of the type of work carried out.

University of London.   Much of the important work in immunology is centred in London at the myriad of colleges, mostly medical, that constitute the University of London. A particularly active group is working at **University College** in the Tumour Immunology Unit of the Department of Zoology, which is solely financed and run by the Imperial Cancer Research Fund. Their work includes regulation of the immune response using allo- and viral antigens, characterization of T-cells using monoclonal antibodies, and studying T-cell-mediated suppressor activity. The **Royal Postgraduate Medical School** carries out immunological research in three departments: Haematology, Medicine (which houses the MRC Clinical Immunology Research Group) and Immunology. Activities include immunosuppression and bone marrow transplantation, surface markers in leukaemia, immunopathology, and asthma.

The **Middlesex Hospital** Medical School's Department of Immunology has a large programme of research which includes: rheumatoid arthritis and other aspects of autoimmunity; vaccines based on monoclonal antibody anti-idiotypes; and enhancement of the immune response by IgM monoclonal antibodies.

The **Cardiothoracic Institute** carries out a large number of projects, mainly in the area of respiratory allergies and neutrophil chemotaxis, in its Department of Allergy and Clinical Immunology.

At the **King's College Hospital** Medical School, the Department of Immunology and the Liver Unit carry out research into the immunology of both acute and chronic hepatitis, and work on the hormonal control of the immune response in cancer.

The Bone and Joint Research Unit at the **London Hospital** Medical College are involved in rheumatoid arthritis research.

Also the following London colleges are of some interest: **St Mary's,** with its work on SLE and multiple sclerosis; **St Thomas's,** for work on lymphoproliferative disease; and the **Institute of Child Health,** for paediatric immunology.

Provincial and Scottish Universities. An extensive immunological research programme is run at the **University of Glasgow.** It is shared between the

Department of Bacteriology and Immunology, the Department of Pathology, the Department of Neurology, the Department of Infectious Diseases and the Veterinary School. The work includes: isolation and characterization of gut mucosal lymphocytes; behaviour and adhesion of lymphocytes; immune complex; and immunology of feline leukaemias.

There is an MRC Cellular Immunology Unit associated with the **Sir William Dunn School of Pathology** at Oxford, whose activities cover the serology of legionella species, and the properties and roles of antigens on the surface of lymphocytes.

The work of the Immunobiology Group at the **University of Bristol**'s Department of Pathology includes the immunological characterization of glomerular basement membrane antigens, the immunology of Epstein–Barr virus and the immunological control of animal growth.

At the **University of Manchester,** immunological research is shared by two departments: the Department of Clinical Rheumatism, with its associated Rheumatism Research Centre, and the Department of Immunology. The work includes studies of the effect of gold in rheumatoid arthritis, and lymphocyte and humoral abnormalities in connective tissue disorders.

The Department of Immunology at the Medical School of the **University of Birmingham** has a diverse research programme; tumour immunology, viral immunology (in collaboration with the Department of Medical Microbiology), and the problems of 'scaling-up' in hybridoma technology.

At the **University of Cambridge,** the Department of Pathology carries out research into markers of the major histocompatibility system in transplantation and disease.

Parasite immunology is a speciality of the Department of Zoology at the **University of Nottingham.** Related work is also carried out in the Immunology Department.

Other notable universities include **Southampton** (Department of Immunochemistry) and **Sheffield** (Department of Haematology). Part of the library service at Sheffield is the Biomedical Information Service. BIS provides a monthly current-awareness service in the form of bulletins, the most relevant of which are *Monoclonal Antibodies, Immunoassay* and *Immunohistochemistry*.

Study

Undergraduates generally become acquainted with immunology for the first time when studying medicine, microbiology, biological sciences, biochemistry and, to a limited extent, veterinary sciences. However, a number of BSc courses exist which specify immunology in the title. At **Glasgow** an immunology course is run, although entry is to the Faculty of Science and not to a particular course. Applicants choose a preferred course, but if admitted they have a free choice of courses, subject to approval by the university.

A CNAA BSc (Hons) Immunology, and an MIBiol Immunology, course is run by the **North East Surrey College of Technology.**

Students have a choice of three courses at **Chelsea College** (University of London): immunology with biochemistry, microbiology or physiology. At Aberystwyth, the **University College of Wales** offers a course entitled 'Cell and Immuno-biology'.

There are a number of postgraduate courses, most of which involve carrying out research projects leading to MPhil and PhD degrees, but there are also a number of taught courses leading to an MSc.

For those wishing to study part-time, **Brunel University, Chelsea College,** the **North East London Polytechnic** and **St Thomas's Hospital Medical School** offer two-year MSc courses in immunology. A one-year full-time MSc course is offered by **Birmingham University.**

There are numerous less formal courses for postgraduates. **Chelsea College** provides a post-experience course in immunology, which lasts for three terms. The **Royal Postgraduate Medical School** runs an annual full-time course specializing in the clinical aspects of cellular and molecular immunology. The NELP runs three very well established courses: Cellular Immunology, Techniques, and a Radio Immunoassay Intensive Course. These courses concentrate primarily on practical work.

It is possible to carry out an immunologically related PhD project in virtually every university or college in the UK which has a biological or medical department, subject, of course, to having a good honours degree (or equivalent) in a relevant discipline.

The best and most financially attractive method of entry is via studentships; these are generally advertised in *Nature* and *New Scientist.* Many bodies provide grants: the MRC, the SERC, the Wellcome Trust, the AFRC and MAFF. The course of study is specified by the sponsor, and is carried out in a university department over three years. The **British Society of Immunology** holds a register of individuals or departments who are willing to offer research training in immunology leading to PhD.

For the post-doctoral research worker, a number of opportunities exist for research fellowships. The **Wellcome Trust** offers Travelling Research Fellowships, which are normally for one year. The **Royal Society** also sponsors post-doctoral studies. Many universities offer fellowships, which involve a period of research, usually not more than two years, on a particular topic.

Private research institutes

In the UK the only major privately funded research institutes are those run by the cancer societies.

The Cancer Research Campaign provides the largest support for research into all forms of cancer. Of its total expenditure of nearly £20 million in 1982, just under half went to university research. A third went in support of research at the Beatson Institute, Glasgow; the Institute of Cancer Research, London; the Paterson Laboratories; and the CRC's own Gray Laboratory. The rest was spent on providing new laboratory facilities in medical schools and universities, fellowships, and support for meetings. General immunology is practised at all the laboratories mentioned, although mainly in the area of tumour immunology. Campaign-funded research into the clinical aspects of monoclonal antibodies is taking place in 11 establishments, foremost of which are the University of Birmingham, the University of Nottingham and the John Radcliffe Hospital, Oxford.

The Imperial Cancer Research Fund has three main laboratories; the world-famous Institute at Lincoln's Inn Fields, and smaller laboratories at Mill Hill (London) and Edinburgh. Three extramural units, at St Bartholomew's Hospital, Guy's Hospital and University College London, carry out many of the clinical trials organized by the Fund. It also provides funds for studentships, postdoctoral fellowships, and grants for research.

3.6 NATIONAL ORGANIZATIONS — USA
Associations

American Association for Clinical Immunology and Allergy

The American Association for Clinical Immunology and Allergy (AACIA) was founded in 1964. It has about 1100 members, who are practising allergists and immunologists. Its aims are to encourage the study, improve the practice and advance the cause of clinical immunology and allergy. The Association comprises five committees: Education, Ethics, Program, Publications, and Research. Awards are presented to selected fellows in the field and in 'specialized continuing medical education'. Amongst the Association's publications are: *Immunology and Allergy Practice*, which is a bimonthly journal; a newsletter, which is also bimonthly; and a biennial *Roster,* containing members' names and addresses, etc. The Association meets annually (in 1984 the meeting was held in Palm Springs, California) with lectures and a Continuing Medical Education course. The Association is affiliated to the American Board of Allergy and Immunology, and has links with the International Association of Allergology.

American Association of Immunologists

The American Association of Immunologists (AAI) is the oldest, largest and most important of the national immunological societies. It was founded in 1914, and today has a membership of over 3000. Its members are scientists from many disciplines (including virology, biochemistry and bacteriology) engaged in immunological research. The AAI is noted for its monthly publication *Journal of Immunology* — certainly the most prestigious immunology journal. Also, a newsletter is circulated among members three times a year. The Association is composed of seven committees: Awards, Clinical Immunology, Education, IUIS Advisory, Minority Group Immunology, Standardization, and Status of Women. Its annual convention is held with the Federation of American Societies for Experimental Biology. The Association was a founding member of the IUIS.

American Board of Allergy and Immunology

The American Board of Allergy and Immunology (ABAI), founded in 1972, is run jointly by the American Board of Internal Medicine and the American Board of Pediatrics. It is an academic body (for internists and paediatricians with special competency in allergic and immunological problems) which establishes qualifications and examines candidates for certification as specialists in allergy and immunology. The ABAI is affiliated to the American Academy of Allergy, which publishes the *Journal of Allergy and Clinical Immunology*, and the American Association for Clinical Immunology and Allergy.

American Board of Clinical Immunology and Allergy

The American Board of Clinical Immunology and Allergy (ABCIA) promotes continuing education for clinical allergists, conducts an active research programme, and sponsors semi-annual major postgraduate education programmes. It was founded in 1964 and boasts 1100 members who meet annually; the 1984 meeting was in Palm Springs. It is affiliated to the AACIA.

American Dermatologic Society of Allergy and Immunology

The American Dermatologic Society of Allergy and Immunology has a small specialist membership of 150 members, who are mostly physicians who run a practice covering dermatology, allergy and immunology. Its purpose is largely educational, and its main activity is the annual preparation of a postgraduate course. The Society presents the Marion Sulzberg Award for leaders in immunological research, usually at its annual convention held in September.

Foundation for Cure

The Foundation for Cure has a very impressive set of objectives, among which are: to provide funds for research in immunology; to provide hospitals for patients with clinical immunological problems; to provide a laboratory for reagent and vaccine production, and to correlate clinical and immunochemistry. How far the Foundation has achieved its aims since its inception in 1969 is uncertain. It has a small publishing programme which includes *Patient's manual of clinical immunology*, *Antigens and why* and other medical books.

American Association for Tissue Banks

The main concerns of the American Association for Tissue Banks are the development of regional tissue banks and the establishment of guidelines and standards for the collection, preservation, distribution and use of tissue for transplantation. The Association, which was founded in 1976, is divided into the following councils: musculo-skeletal, ocular, renal, reproductive, skin, and tissue bank. It publishes a quarterly newsletter and guidelines for tissue processing.

Government bodies

National Institutes of Health

The National Institutes of Health (NIH) are the principal agencies of the Department of Health for promoting biomedical research, research training and biomedical communication in the interests of public health. The NIH also provide the major funds for research in the universities and institutes. In 1984 the NIH were granted a total of $4.3 billion by Congress to carry out their many and varied duties: cancer studies, environmental health services, general medical sciences, supporting the Library of Medicine and (the most relevant to the discussion here) allergy and infectious disease.

The NIH comprise 12 institutes, nearly half of which carry out some immunological research. Most of the NIH institutes are located in a giant complex at Bethesda, Maryland.

The **National Institute of Allergy and Infectious Disease** (NIAID) is, perhaps, the most important institute in terms of immunological activity; it receives about 14% of the entire NIH budget, of which $29 million has been set aside for AIDS research. Its aims are: solving new problems in allergic diseases; tackling unsolved problems in bacterial diseases; and, more generally, developing a useful body of knowledge relating to viral diseases. The NIAID is divided into a number of laboratories, which themselves are divided into sections. The Laboratory of Immunology carries out a comprehensive programme of research into such topics as B-cell growth factors and T-cell antigen receptors; the Laboratory of Immunogenetics is investigating insulin-specific T-cell hybridomas; the Laboratory of Microbial Immunity is concerned with various aspects of parasitic immunology, and autoimmunity; and the Laboratory of Clinical Investigation covers lymphocyte blastogenesis and complement activation.

The **National Cancer Institute** (NCI) broadly supports research into the causes, detection, diagnosis and treatment of cancer. Its work is shared amongst a number of branches. The Immunology Branch conducts work on the major histo-compatibility complex, NK-derived T-cells, and human T-cell lymphocyte clones, mainly in its Laboratory of Cell Biology. Other branches of importance are: Pediatric Oncology, Environmental Epidemiology, Dermatology, and Metabolism. As well as the Bethesda Laboratory, the NCI also has the Frederick Cancer Research Facility, which contains the Laboratory of Tumor Immunology and Biology. The nature of its work is reflected in the names of the sections, which are: molecular mechanisms of T-cell leukemogenesis, immunochemistry, natural immunity, and cellular and molecular physiology.

The **National Institute of Arthritis, Diabetes, Digestion and Kidney Diseases** (NIADDKD) carries out a great deal of work on autoimmunity, mainly in the cellular immunology section of the Arthritis and Rheumatism Branch.

The **National Institute of Dental Research**'s programme of immunological research is conducted in the Laboratory of Microbiology and Immunology. Examples of its work include research into immune interferon, and lymphokine-stimulating monocytes.

The Neuroimmunology Branch of the **National Institute of Neurological and Communicative Disorders and Stroke** and the Laboratory of Molecular Genetics of the **National Institute of Child Health and Human Development** have a small immunological research programme.

Private research institutes

The private research institutes have always been a force in American scientific research, but the last 10 years has witnessed a significant increase both in their numbers and the influence they are having, particularly in the areas of hybridoma and recombinant DNA technology. In most cases they have been funded by foundations such as those of Rockefeller and Howard Hughes, multinational companies like Hoffman-La Roche, or by charitable bodies inter-ested in cancer and arthritis research. Their aim is to promote ideas which, it is hoped, will result in the development of new products that will be commercially valuable. The status of the institutes — as tax-deductable charitable organiza-tions — has also made them somewhat attractive to the multi-billion dollar corporations. But it should be added that, in most cases, the academic freedom of these 'centres of excellence' is guaranteed.

Measured in terms of publishing output, the Scripps Clinic and Research Foundation (partly funded by Eli Lilly) is the most active of them, publishing prolifically in the *Journal of Immunology* and *Immunology*. Such has been the success of the Foundation in the field of immunochemistry that it recently formed a new company with Miles Laboratory Inc., to undertake large-scale production of immuno-chemicals, including monoclonal antibodies. The research activities of the Foundation, carried out in the Departments of Immunopathology and Basic Clinical Research in La Jolla, cover immunodeficiency diseases, kidney immunopathology, IgE formation *in vitro* and macrophage activation. The Foundation collaborates widely with universities, such as North Western in Chicago.

The Wistar Institute in Philadelphia is noted for its pioneering work in hybridoma technology — it scored a first with its reporting of the production of human monoclonal antibodies. The Institute has ties with Centocor Inc., a firm interested in the diagnostic applications of monoclonals. Recent research by the Institute includes investigations on influenza-specific cytotoxic lymphocytes, retroviral envelope antigens, and granulocyte surface antigens.

The Salk Institute, like the Wistar, is a leader in the field of hybridoma technology and is also active in the field of tumour immunology.

The Howard Hughes Medical Institute Laboratories, which are on the campus of the University of California at San Francisco, conduct an extensive immunological research programme in collaboration with the University. Fields of interest include human T-cell stimulation and receptors of monocytes, B-cells and non B-cells. The work is mainly carried out in the Department of Cellular Immunology.

A number of cancer institutes carry out work on tumour immunology, as well as basic immunology. These include the Fred Hutchinson Cancer Research Center, the Michigan Cancer Foundation, and the Sidney and Dana Farber Cancer Institutes — the last being part of the Harvard Medical School.

Close relationships also exist between other institutes and universities: the Palo Alto Medical Foundation and the Stanford Medical School; the Molecular Biology Institute and UCLA: the Mayo Clinic and the Mayo Medical School in Rochester.

Universities and colleges

Spending on basic research by universities and colleges has risen dramatically from less than $200 million in 1953 to more than $1600 million in 1981. In contrast, spending by industry has remained roughly constant since 1960, at about $215 million. University research in immunology is funded almost exclusively by the government, in the form of grants from the various institutes that comprise the NIH, NIAID, NCI and NIADDKD. Other sources of financial support include the American Cancer Society, the National Science Foundation, the Arthritis Foundation and the Rockefeller Foundation.

It is not possible to describe comprehensively the activities of all the universities and medical colleges where immunological research is undertaken, because of their sheer number — on the evidence of the papers published in the *Journal of Immunology* over one hundred carry out some kind of advanced immunological research.

Some indication of the relative strengths of the various universities — in the absence of an up-to-date guide to research in the USA — can be gauged by a recent survey conducted by the National Academy of Sciences in 1983. Entitled 'An assessment of research doctorate programs in the United States: biological sciences' it asked 2000 academic biologists to rate programmes in terms of the quality of their faculty and their effectiveness in educating graduate students; only 56% of those asked agreed to participate in this subjective exercise. The two areas of biology specifically mentioned were cell and molecular biology, and microbiology — disciplines which are closely bound with immunology. The

Table 3.4   Relative strengths of US universities in biology

Cell/molecular biology	Microbiology
1 Massachusetts Institute of Technology	1 Massachusetts Institute of Technology
2 California Institute of Technology	2 California Institute of Technology
3 Rockefeller	3 Washington at Seattle
4 Yale	4 Johns Hopkins
5 Wisconsin–Madison	5 California, San Diego
6 Harvard	6 Chicago
7 California, San Diego	7 Pennsylvania (immunology)
8 California, Berkeley	8 Duke
9 Columbia	9 California, Los Angeles
10 Colorado	10 Columbia
11 Stanford	11 Stanford
12 Washington at Seattle	

Source: *An assessment of research doctorate programs in the United States: biological sciences* by the National Academy of Sciences, Washington, D.C., 1983.

results, in rank order, are shown in *Table 3.4*. Those colleges figuring highly under both disciplines were the Massachusetts Institute of Technology (MIT); Rockefeller; Washington at Seattle; California at San Diego; Columbia; and Stanford. Pennsylvania was singled out specifically for its immunology.

Our own assessment of the leading universities in immunology was based on a quantitative analysis of papers published in the *Journal of Immunology*, and theses recorded in *Dissertation Abstracts International*. From such sources it was possible to identify 20 universities which we felt were making a major specialist contribution to the field. (A surprising degree of correlation occurred between our survey and that carried out by the National Academy of Sciences, with 14 universities featuring in both.) They are listed in order of importance, first by name of university and the interested department(s), followed by an indication of its subject specialities.

1. Harvard Medical School: Department of Medicine (autoreactive T-cell clones, haematopoietic ontogeny, monoclonal antibodies to *Leishmania*, auto-antibodies to native DNA); Department of Pathology (hapten-specific T-cell immunity, aspects of immunosuppression); Department of Genetics (aspects of immunogenetics).

Harvard collaborates extensively with Brigham and Women's Hospital, and with the Dana and Sidney Farber Cancer Institutes of Boston.

2. Johns Hopkins University School of Medicine: Department of Medicine (mucosal immunity, mast cell mediators); Department of Pharmacology and Experimental Therapeutics (granulocyte surface antigens); Department of Physiological Chemistry (1a antigens).

It collaborates with the Good Samaritan Hospital and Baltimore City Hospitals.

3. University of Washington School of Medicine at Seattle: Department of Medicine (human suppressor T-cells); Department of Microbiology and Immunology (natural killer cell immunity).

The Fred Hutchinson Cancer Research Center is located at the university.

4. Stanford University School of Medicine: Department of Pathology (thymus-homing bone marrow cells, T-cell proliferation); Department of Structural Biology (monoclonal antibody production and proliferation).

5. University of Chicago: Departments of Pediatrics and Pathology (T-cells: proliferation and suppression); Department of Biochemistry and the Committee on Immunology (biological properties of T-cell growth factors).

6. University of Alabama in Birmingham: Departments of Microbiology and Pathology, the Comprehensive Cancer Center (IgA responses in mice); Cellular Immunology Unit, Tumor Institute, Department of Pediatrics (T-cell suppression and proliferation).

7. University of Texas Health Science Center at Dallas: Departments of Ophthalmology, Cell Biology and Internal Medicine (suppression of delayed-type hypersensitivity); Departments of Pathology and Microbiology (natural killer cells).

8. Yale University School of Medicine: Section of Clinical Immunology and Allergy, Department of Medicine (delayed-type hypersensitivity); Department of Epidemiology and Public Health (delayed-type hypersensitivity).

9. University of Colorado Health Sciences Center: Departments of Pathology and Medicine (B-cell activation, anti-histone antibodies); Division of Clinical Immunology; Department of Microbiology/Immunology (delayed-type hypersensitivity).

10. University of California, San Diego: Department of Pediatrics (immunodeficiency diseases); Departments of Pathology and Surgery (various aspects of tumour immunology); Department of Medicine (T-cell deficiency in listeriosis).

11. Columbia University College of Physicians and Surgeons: Department of Pathology (anti-idiotypic antibodies).

12. University of Michigan Medical School: Department of Microbiology and Immunology (immune response gene function).

13. University of Pennsylvania School of Medicine: Division of Research Immunology, Department of Pathology and Laboratory Medicine (T-cell subsets in allergic encephalomyelitis).

14. Duke University Medical Center: Department of Medicine (Fc receptors); Departments of Microbiology, Immunology and Surgery (protein antigenicity); Division of Immunology (monocyte and tumour cell interaction).

15. North Western University Medical School: Department of Microbiology and Immunology (induction and regulation of helper T-cells, idiotype suppression).

16. State University of New York at Buffalo: Department of Microbiology and Oral Pathology (immunization against dental caries).

17. University of California School of Medicine, Davis: Department of Medical Microbiology and Immunology (various aspects of immunogenetics).

18. University of California School of Medicine, Los Angeles: Departments of Medicine, and Microbiology and Immunology (natural killer cell mechanism, monocyte Fc receptors in SLE).

19. Rockefeller University: Laboratory of Cellular Physiology and Immunology (macrophage antimicrobial activity).

20. Massachusetts Institute of Technology: Department of Biology (interferon-mediated induction of antigen presentation).

3.7 NATIONAL ORGANIZATIONS — AUSTRALIA

The Federal government directly funds and conducts research through the National Health, Medical Research Council and the Commonwealth Scientific and Industrial Research Organization (CSIRO). It indirectly supports research through grants to universities and special departmental institutions and laboratories.

CSIRO accounts for 40% of all aid to biology. Its main role is to plan and execute a programme of general scientific research, which it does with a staff of over 7000 employed in laboratories throughout the country. It also trains, makes grants and awards, and liaises with other countries in matters of scientific research.

CSIRO's immunological research takes place mostly under the aegis of the Institute of Animal and Food Sciences, at a number of laboratories. The Molecular and Cellular Biology Unit at North Ryde has developed immunoassay kits, using monoclonal antibodies against a series of human hormones. Other areas where monoclonal antibodies are being used include hepatitis, detection of food spoilage antigen (in collaboration with CSIRO, Sydney) and in the study of influenza viruses. The Australian National Animal Health Laboratory was to have been a centre for vaccine production, as well as providing high-risk disease containment; some uncertainty over its function prevails at the present time.

The National Biological Standards Laboratory at Canberra, which is part of the Department of Health, is a control authority for medical and veterinary vaccines.

Prominent among the research institutes is the Walter and Elisa Hall Institute of Medical Research, which is part of the Royal Melbourne Hospital. The Immunoregulation Laboratory collaborates with the Ludwig Cancer Institute on aspects of cellular immunity. Experimental Allergy and Cancer Research Units are also found in the Hospital. The Immunology Unit of the Kanematsu Memorial Institute at the Sydney Hospital researches into aspects of T-cell immunity and photoimmunology.

Universities active in the field of immunology research and education include the University of Sydney, which contains the Clinical Immunology Research Centre, and the Departments of Microbiology and Immunology at the John Curtin School of Medical Research belonging to the Australian National University. The University also houses the Australian Society for Immunology. The Society was one of the founder members of the IUIS, and has just under 400 members.

3.8 NATIONAL ORGANIZATIONS — CANADA

Direct government involvement in scientific research is largely confined to the Department of Agriculture although, of course, the government does provide much of the funding for research in the universities and hospitals via the Medical Research Council. The part devoted by the MRC to immunological research projects in 1978 was about 7% of the total grant budget.

The universities generate most of the immunological research in Canada. Some of the most active are listed, with an indication of the nature of their work in parentheses.

The Institut Armand Frappier (viral immunity) and the Institute of Microbiology and Hygiene (general immunology), both of the University of Montreal; the Ontario Cancer Institute and Institute of Immunology (tumour immunology and general immunology), both of the University of Toronto; Rheumatic Disease Research Laboratories (immunoregulation) and the MRC Group for Allergic Research (IgE responses) at the University of Manitoba; the Department of Immunology, University of Alberta (lymphoproliferative disorders); and the Department of Anatomy, McGill University (transplantation).

Merck Frosst Canada Inc. leads the commercial interest in immunology in Canada. Much of its work is devoted to allergic asthma.

The Canadian professional body is the Canadian Society for Immunology, which has approximately 360 members. It was one of the founder members of the IUIS.

3.9 NATIONAL ORGANIZATIONS — FRANCE

The Ministry of Research and Technology finances science through two large research organizations or 'grands organismes'. They are the CNRS (Centre National de la Recherche Scientifique) and INSERM (Institut National de la Santé et de la Recherche Médicale).

The CNRS is the larger of the two bodies, receiving nearly a third of the scientific budget — just under F6000 million in 1981. It employs 23 000 people, of whom 9000 are research staff distributed in 1200 laboratories throughout the country, although only 150 are fully controlled by CNRS; 250 are shared with the universities, and the rest co-run with INSERM and hospitals.

INSERM supports 1500 researchers, and is the largest employer of French biologists. It received just over F1000 million in 1981.

Immunological research is carried out at a great many centres in France; the most important is the Centre d'Immunologie at Marseille, which is jointly run by INSERM and the CNRS. It carries out a large programme of research in immunology, and is most noted for its work on the major histocompatibility complex. First refusal rights on some of INSERM's immunological research have been granted to the commercial company Immunotech, whose laboratory is adjacent to the Centre d'Immunologie. The Institut Pasteur in Paris is linked to 26 similar institutes around the world. It has played a leading role in hybridoma technology and AIDS research, and has recently developed a vaccine against hepatitis B infection. The Institut Pasteur in Lille boasts a Centre d'Immunologie et de Biologie Parasitaire where the immunology of parasitic infections is studied. The Institut de Recherches Scientifiques sur le Cancer at Villejuif conducts basic research in immunopathology, cellular immunology and tumour immunology, in its Laboratory of Cellular Immunology. Work of a similar nature is carried out at the Laboratoire d'Immunopharmacologie des Tumeurs, Montpellier, the Laboratoire d'Immunologie et de Virologie des Tumeurs at the Hôpital Cochin in Paris, and at the Centre Léon Berard in Lyon. Problems of a more exotic nature, including research on the immune response of fish, are investigated at the Laboratoire d'Immunologie Comparée.

The welfare of French immunologists is the responsibility of the Société Française d'Immunologie at the Institut Pasteur and the Société Française d'Allergologie.

3.10 NATIONAL ORGANIZATIONS — FEDERAL REPUBLIC OF GERMANY

West Germany spends more money on research than any other country in Europe, most of the money being spent by the German universities. There is a single agency for supporting research in the higher-educational establishment: the Deutsche Forschungsgemeinschaft (German Research Society). It is not a government agency but more akin to the operating charities in the UK, or the 'not for profit' organizations in the USA. The Society consists of a collection of legally autonomous academic institutions — mainly universities, but there are also some national research organizations. Of the DM900 million it was granted in 1981, about 38% was spent on biology (including medicine).

The following universities play a leading role in the various aspects of immunological research. Some indication of their activities is given in parentheses: the Institute of Medical Microbiology, University of Johannes Gutenberg (complement); the Institute of Physiology, University of Marburg (neuroimmunology); the Institute of Clinical Immunology and Blood Transfusion, University of Giessen (reproductive immunology); the Department of Immunology, University of Munster (cellular immunity); the Institute of Genetics, University of Cologne (immunogenetics); and the Centre for Medical Microbiology and Immunology, Ruhr University (microbial immunity).

The Max-Planck-Gesellschaft zur Förderung der Wissenschaften EV (Max Planck Society for Advancement of Science) is an internationally renowned research organization which comprises 49 institutes scattered throughout the country. The Max Planck Institute for Immunology, Freiburg, and the Max Planck Institute for Biology, Tübingen, are the most relevant to immunology.

Heidelberg is the major (and overcrowded) centre for biomedical research in Germany. It houses on one science park the European Molecular Biology Organization (EMBO), the Institute of Immunology and Genetics, the Cancer Research Centre, and the University of Heidelberg's Institute of Immunology and Serology. In 1984 the university acquired a new institute for molecular biology started by grants from the chemical giant BASF. A further development at Heidelberg is the formation of a small biotechnology company Progen Biotechnik, which began producing antibody-based diagnostic kits recently.

The Gesellschaft für Immunologie looks after the interests of immunologists in West Germany. The Society, one of the founder members of IUIS, has almost 700 members.

.11 NATIONAL ORGANIZATIONS — JAPAN

Immunological research in Japan today is as advanced as anywhere in the world, as *Figure 3.1* confirms. This is partly because so many of its immunologists have worked abroad, mainly in the USA, but also in Europe, and have now taken this expertise home; the links forged as a consequence of this interaction are evident in the many collaborative research programmes between the West and Japan. The main bulk of this research is carried out in the 800 universities and colleges in Japan today. Unlike those in the West, the activities of the Japanese colleges have scarcely been impeded by the worldwide recession.

Initially, research was financed by government grant-in-aid on a three-year basis. This was so successful that it was extended for a further three years. Now immunology has established its right to continuous support, through funds allocated to pathology.

It is impossible to mention all the colleges and institutes where immunological research takes place: the activities of the main centres only will be described briefly.

The Institute for Molecular and Cellular Biology was recently established in Osaka University, to investigate homoeostatic mechanisms that prevent disease in man. The Institute for Medical Immunology at Kumamoto University Medical School is particularly active in the fields of immunochemistry and clinical immunology. Cellular immunology is a specialism of research conducted by the Department of Immunology at Tokyo University, which incidentally is the oldest of its type in Japan, having been founded in 1918 as the Department of Serology. The government's National Institute of Health in Tokyo has a special interest in immunity to infectious disease. The University at Hokkaido is one of the world's centres for HLA research and has also played an important role in the investigation of rat MHC. The Aichi Cancer Center and the National Cancer Center are working on various aspects of tumour immunology. Osaka University Hospital has been one of the pioneers in hybridoma technology.

The Japanese Society for Immunologists was founded in 1971, and today has 2500 members. The Japanese Society of Allergology, a smaller, more specialized association, was founded in 1950. The Japanese Society of Clinical Immunology, which was established in 1972, is principally aimed at medical practitioners and those in hospital laboratories.

A more comprehensive account of immunology in Japan can be found in a supplement of *Immunology Today* (June 1983) which was published to coincide with the 5th International Congress in Immunology held in Kyoto in 1983. It includes the names and addresses of over one hundred leading Japanese immunologists.

.12 NATIONAL ORGANIZATIONS —SWITZERLAND

The National Science Foundation, a nominally private institution, supports most basic science in Switzerland, which incidentally spends more on research and development, per head of population, than any other country in the world. Research effort is evenly divided amongst government, university, private institutes and industry, although in terms of total spending three-quarters is spent by industry, making Switzerland unique.

Entirely supported by the pharmaceutical giant F. Hoffman-La Roche, the Basel Institute of Immunology may justly claim to be the foremost centre of immunological research in the world. It was founded in 1968 and began operations in 1971. Ten years later 130 staff— evenly divided between scientists and technicians (only these two grades exist) — conduct more than one hundred research projects and collaborate with scientists working in Canada, Denmark, Finland, the UK, the Netherlands, Sweden and the USA.

The productivity of the Institute can be gauged by the fact that between 1980 and 1981 a total of 227 papers or books were published by members; 75 formal seminars were given at the Institute; and members contributed to nearly 200 symposia meetings, seminars, or courses held worldwide.

The international reputation of the Institute is such that 40 'visiting' immunologists spent some time there in 1981.

It would be impossible comprehensively to describe the range of work of the Institute as it covers the entire immunology spectrum and the following species: mice, humans, rats, sheep, chickens and frogs. Most projects concern differentiation, factors active on lymphocytes, MCA and somatic cell genetics, helper T-cells and T–B collaboration, cytotoxic and alloreactive T-cells, and lymphocyte cell surface antigens.

The leading universities are those of Lausanne, Zürich, Basel and Geneva.

The Swiss Institute for Experimental Cancer Research, Epalinges, investigates aspects of tumour immunology.The Swiss Serum and Vaccine Institute, Berne, is concerned with developments in vaccine standardization. Other important institutes include the Institute of Clinical Immunology, Berne, and the Sandoz Research Institute, Zürich.

The Schweizerische Gesellschaft für Allergie und Immunologie was one of the founder members of IUIS and today has 240 members.

Switzerland is also the home of the WHO, which has its headquarters in Geneva. The WHO Immunology Research and Training Centre is located in the complex.

3.13 NATIONAL ORGANIZATIONS — OTHER COUNTRIES

Immunological research in the Netherlands is largely the domain of the universities: the University of Nijmegen (immunoregulation by monoclonal antibodies); the State University of Utrecht (basic immunology); and Erasmus University in Rotterdam (cellular immunology). Contributions are also made by the Central Laboratory for Blood Transfusion (immunohaematology and autoimmunity) and the Netherlands Cancer Institute (cytotoxicity and T-cell differentiation). The Vereniging voor Immunologie is the professional society for Dutch immunologists; it has nearly 800 members, and was one of the founder members of the IUIS.

The contribution made to immunology by the Scandinavians has increased enormously over the last decade; this contribution is shared equally between the government and universities. The leading centres are Uppsala University (microbial immunity), the University of Lund (eosinophil granules), the Karolinska Institute, Stockholm (ontogeny and tumour immunology), and the Institute of Immunology and Rheumatology and the National Hospital, both in Oslo (transplantation). The Scandinavian Society for Immunology has over 700 members, and was one of the founder members of the IUIS.

In Finland, researchers at the University of Turku frequently publish papers in the quality journals, mainly in the area of cellular immunity.

The number of Italian biomedical papers has risen by a quarter since 1980; three-quarters of them are written by university researchers. The leading universities include the University of Padua, the University of Milan and the Centre of Immunology in Rome. Other important institutes include the Sclavo Research Centre, which has research facilities for studying MCA and lymphokines, and the Institute of Pharmacological Research, Mario Negri. Immunologists' interests are looked after by the Societa Italiana di Immunologia ed Immunopatologia, which has 420 members.

Israeli biomedical research is dominated by the world-famous Weizmann Institute of Science, Rehovot. The Department of Cell Biology is the most prolific in immunology. It carries out work on T-cell hybridoma, interferon, auto-immunity and aspects of tumour immunology. The Israel Immunology Society, which is based at the Weizmann Institute, has just over 200 members. It was a founder member of the IUIS.

Poland has a fine record in immunological research, the main contributors being the Institute of Immunology and the Department of Experimental and Clinical Immunology at the Copernicus Medical School in Cracow, and the Institute of Immunology and Experimental Therapeutics in Cracow. The Polish Immunological Society is housed at the Department of Immunology and Rheumatology in Poznan, and is one of the founder members of the IUIS.

4 Immunology: its conferences

4.1 INTRODUCTION

Conferences, congresses, convocations, conventions, symposia, meetings and workshops are, in most cases, different terms for the same thing: a periodic gathering of like-minded individuals meeting to discuss a single topic or a number of related ones. Over the last decade, however, the terms have come to be used by the societies and other groups to indicate the relative importance of their gatherings. Thus a convocation, conference or congress is usually the main gathering held every four years, if the organizing society is international, or annually if it is a national society. The topics discussed will be wide-ranging, and may extend over four or five days. Symposia are more regular events occurring perhaps three or four times a year, and may concentrate on a single topic. Meetings are, by and large, more informal and represent the activities of sub-groups of a society. The term 'workshop' has come to be frequently used to emphasize the detailed and practical nature of the gathering; workshops are also, very often, highly specialized. Meetings and workshops, which seldom last longer than a day, may be held separately but more often they are an accessory to a larger gathering, such as a conference.

In the last few years there has been a spectacular rise in the number of conferences, congresses, etc. in immunology. This has come about for two main reasons. First, the growth and interest in the subject has spawned numerous groups and societies, all anxious to organize discussions on the latest developments. (The January 1984 issue of *Immunology Today* listed a total of nearly 30 conferences organized for the first half of the year.) Secondly, and this is true for science in general, conferences have become big business; a testament to this is the many commercial sponsors and companies founded solely for the purpose of organizing meetings. Meetings organized by commercial interests are usually characterized by large and, at times, exorbitant attendance fees (the size of the fee certainly doesn't correlate with the standing of the speakers, or the quality of the papers).

A recent trend at conferences has been for manufacturers, in return for providing financial assistance to the organizers, to be allowed to exhibit their range of scientific equipment and reagents for the duration of the meeting.

At their best, conferences provide the opportunity for workers in the field to give details of their latest research findings much earlier than would be the case in print; they provide an opportunity for the audience to obtain information on experimental methods that usually are absent from scientific papers and they enable the validity of statements or conclusions made by the speakers to be questioned. It is questionable whether the most fruitful discussions take place in the lecture theatre or informally afterwards. At their worst, conferences can be cliquey, self-congratulatory and unoriginal; it is not unusual for a speaker to give the same paper at maybe three or four different meetings. In addition, because of the specialist nature of immunological research, most of the papers given at a conference will largely be irrelevant to the individual delegate. The widespread use of audiovisual facilities has tended to alleviate the age-old problem of bad speakers, and a summary of the papers is usually provided by the organizers beforehand. One further development at conferences is the appearance of poster sessions which are designed to increase the scientific content of meetings without increasing their duration. The posters are a means of presenting data in a clear and ordered fashion. Delegates have the opportunity to scan the posters before or after the formal sessions.

4.2 GUIDES TO FORTHCOMING CONFERENCES

Once a researcher becomes an established member of the immunological community he or she will have little difficulty in keeping informed of forthcoming conferences. In many cases the researcher will be automatically circulated with details (especially if he or she is a regular attender) and sometimes asked to attend, or even requested to give a paper. Others can obtain the information by scanning the advertisements, or diary, or notes, sections of the relevant journals, most notably:

> *Immunology Today*
> *British Society for Immunology Newsletter*
> *American Association of Immunology Newsletter*
> *Immunology*
> *Journal of Immunology*
> *Journal of Immunological Methods*
> *Immunological Communications*

The larger and most important conferences will also be advertised in *Nature*, *Science*, and *The Lancet*. Generally speaking, notice of a conference is given some 9–12 months prior to the event.

For those requiring a more comprehensive picture, those weary of relying upon the fruits of serendipity alone, and those seeking conferences outside their particular field of expertise, there are specialist tools, albeit published at the general scientific level, that are solely devoted to the listing of forthcoming meetings. Three such lists deserve special mention. *Forthcoming International Scientific and Technical Conferences* is a quarterly journal published by Aslib. Details provided for each conference include date, title, location and organizer/contact. The subject index lists immunology conferences. However, as it is based on keywords in the conference title, it is necessary to search a number of terms (e.g. hybridoma, monoclonal antibodies, lymphocyte). This can be a long job and there is no way of being sure that all the meetings have been found. There is also an alphabetical index to geographical locations and organizations. Searching under the latter for known immunological organizations can improve the precision of the subject search. In the most recent year surveyed (1983) six immunological meetings were publicized in all, with the period of notice varying between six and nine months.

Possibly the most elaborate and comprehensive listings are offered by the two sister publications: *World Meetings outside the United States and Canada* and *World Meetings: United States and Canada*. Published by the Technical Meetings Information Service, the two publications provide a detailed two-year registry of future medical, scientific and technical meetings. Both are quarterly and have exactly the same format; they are divided into two sections: (1) date section and (2) index section. The first section arranges conferences chronologically (in quarters) and provides the following additional details for each: name, headquarters, location, sponsor, contact, technical content of meeting, estimated attendance and any restriction thereon, availability of abstracts or papers, exhibitions, deadlines for submissions. The index section provides access via keyword (up to five awarded), date of meeting, location, sponsor, and deadline for paper or abstract. The January 1984 issues contained details of approximately six immunology conferences, most being notified six months prior to their occurrence. There is a problem for European subscribers though, as there may be a two to three month delay before the publications arrive in the library, which means, of course, that some conferences will actually have already been held. In the 1983/84 issues of the *World Meetings outside the United States and Canada*, conferences were being held at such widely dispersed venues as Budapest, Rome, Berlin, Kyoto, Marrakesh, London and Athens, demonstrating the worldwide interest in the field. As an example of the kinds of conference listed, the one in Hungary, which was held in September 1984, was titled *Current immunological concepts in rheumatology — immunopathology, genetics and therapy*. One such conference listed in the *World Meetings: US and Canada* volume (January 1984 issue) is the Annual Meeting of the Canadian Society for Immunology held in June 1984. Each issue of the two sister publications is completely reviewed and cumulated, and new additions added, so there is just one look-up point and previous issues may be dispensed with.

4.3 TRACING AND LOCATING CONFERENCE PROCEEDINGS *(see* bibliography entries 35–40)

To help overcome some of the problems of tracing conference proceedings there are a number of guides whose sole function is to list the proceedings that have been published. Most include not only separately published proceedings but also those that appear as part of periodicals. However it should be noted that: (a) many list proceedings and not individual papers, with the notable exceptions of *Conference Papers Index* and *Index to Scientific and Technical Proceedings,* and (b) they contain not the actual publications themselves, or even abstracts of them, but simply sufficient details to enable them to be traced (the British Library's *Index of Conference Proceedings* offers the next best thing: a guaranteed loan, or a photocopy, of the required proceedings).

The *Index of Conference Proceedings Received by the BLL,* though compiled in Britain, is international in coverage. Published monthly and cumulated annually, the *Index* lists the conference proceedings received by the British Library Lending Division, which is generally recognized to have the largest collection of proceedings in the world (it currently receives about 15 000 a year). An 18-year cumulation (1964–78) is available on microfiche, providing in one publication access to over 146 000 conference proceedings, making it the largest bibliography of its kind in the world.

In an attempt to overcome the problems of tracing proceedings the *Index* lists proceedings (alphabetically) by keyword extracted from the title, and sometimes the contents if the title is not sufficiently descriptive. As a consequence each proceedings may be listed several times under a number of different subject headings, thus increasing the chance of its location.

The adoption of an alphabetic subject keyword approach does mean that not all immunological conferences are located together; they are scattered according to the alphabetical position of the words in their titles. A good number (around six per issue) can be found under the root *immun-*, but one also needs to look under allergy, transplantation, monoclonal antibodies, etc.

Most of the immunology proceedings listed in the monthly issues are over a year old, but this may be as much to do with late publication as late acquisition.

The *Index* is also available on-line via BLAISE-Line, and is on the file known as *Conference Proceedings Index*. Over 155 000 conferences are listed on this file, and approximately 850 of these are immunological in content. The file is updated monthly, and can be searched back to 1964. Apart from the speed of search the major advantage of accessing the *Index* via the computer is that it offers the enquirer more search pathways. Thus a search may be conducted on any terms or combination of terms present in the conference's title (not just the keywords), author statement and publication description (date, location, etc.).

The *Index to Scientific and Technical Proceedings*, published monthly by the Institute for Scientific Information (ISI), is a relatively recent newcomer to the field: it was begun in 1978 and is therefore of limited retrospective use. The *Index* lists approximately 3300 proceedings from conferences held around the world, irrespective of language. It claims to cover around half of all proceedings published, and 75–90% of the most significant. Perhaps its major asset is that under each conference (arranged arbitrarily by an ISI accession number) it lists all the authors and titles of the papers submitted — around 112 000 papers are listed in this way. Six indexes provide a variety of approaches to locating proceedings: by category of conference topics (broad subject headings, which include allergy and immunology); by title words of papers, books and conferences; author/editor; sponsor; meeting location and corporate name. About nine immunological conferences are listed in each issue, although of course the number of immunological papers will be far greater as many will be delivered at related subject conferences. Thus monoclonals was the topic at over two dozen papers in a typical monthly issue. Reporting of conferences proceedings is relatively rapid, with the immunology conferences being listed about 6–12 months after the event. What is particularly good about the *Index* is that unlike many of its competitors it actually appears in the month advertised on the cover. Thus January 1984's issue actually arrived on the shelves of British libraries by the end of January. An example of the kind of proceedings covered is the National Symposium on Hybridomas and Cellular Immunology, held in Houston, Texas on 5–6 November 1981. The proceedings were published as a book by Plenum in 1983, and appeared in the *Index* in January 1984, where the seventeen papers delivered at the conference were listed, complete with the authors' names and addresses.

The monthly *Conference Papers Index*, published by Cambridge Scientific Abstracts, provides a classified listing of meetings, which has the merit of permitting browsing. There is a section called 'Biochemistry and biology' where most of the immunology conference proceedings will be found. Under each meeting all the papers that are featured in the published proceedings are listed. Ordering details are also provided. *Conference Proceedings Index* is held on-line on the BRS, DIALOG, and ESA-IRS systems. On DIALOG the file covering the years 1973 to date amounts to over 1 000 000 records. A sample search on conference titles for immunology yielded 3700 records, and one on the index term monoclonal produced 1278 papers. The file is relatively up-to-date with most papers appearing about six months after they were presented at conference. Each record gives the names and addresses of the authors of the papers, publication and ordering details, and announcements of any publications issued at the meeting.

Two other useful specialist print lists are: Interdok's *Directory of Published Proceedings*, a chronologically arranged listing appearing monthly, which is of considerable value to those searching retrospectively as it has been going since 1964. A keyword index provides access to immunological conferences (two being listed in December 1983's issue); and *Proceedings in Print*, which arranges proceedings by accession number. Access to immunology conferences is through the keyword index, where 7 proceedings are listed, most published in 1982 and 1983. Coverage is international; a French proceedings is listed in the August 1983 issue. This semi-annual publication is mainly of value as a guide to purchasing. Currency is a particular problem for European subscribers, issues not arriving until five to six months after their posted date.

The *System for Information on Grey Literature in Europe (SIGLE)*, available through the BLAISE-Line and Inka on-line services, while not exclusively a proceedings source does deserve mention as 25% of the records are of conference contributions — some 6000 papers in all. Coverage is restricted to the European Communities. The file goes back to 1981. Biomedical sciences are listed as one of its subject strengths, and it may be searched, for example, by subject heading, language, country of publication and, perhaps most importantly, by document form, enabling a direct search for conference proceedings. The Inka database is very similar to DIALOG to search, and is updated every two months.

4.4 THE MAJOR IMMUNOLOGY CONFERENCES

It would be virtually impossible to list all the conferences held on immunology or immunologically related topics because of their number and diversity. Many are one-off affairs and will not be considered here; however where their proceedings have been published, reference will be found in section 5.3, 'Books'. In this section only the major, regularly occurring conferences in immunology, allergy and transplantation will be discussed.

International Congresses of Immunology

The Congresses are undoubtedly the highlight of the immunological calendar. The first was held in Washington, D.C., as recently as 1–6 August 1971, and organized under the sponsorship of the IUIS and the American Association of Immunologists. The Congress volume *Progress in Immunology* was published within four months of the Congress. This Congress was attended by 3400 participants representing 45 countries — a very early demonstration of the widespread interest in the field.

The 2nd International Congress of Immunology, organized by the British Society for Immunology, was held in Brighton, 21–26 July 1974. About 4500 delegates attended. The symposia and summaries of the workshops were published in 5 volumes, averaging more than 400 pages each (*Progress in Immunology II*). Twenty-five symposia and 163 workshops were held at the Congress.

Sydney hosted the 3rd International Congress in July 3–8, 1977 at which only 1100 immunologists attended — a result perhaps of the antipodean location. The symposia and reports of workshops are included in *Progress in Immunology III*.

The 4th International Congress was organized by the French Society of Immunology and held in Paris on 21–26 July 1980. Over 5000 people attended the Congress; 4000 abstracts were accepted for presentation, 2800 of which were presented on posters. The programme was organized around 20 teams, each composed of a symposium and eight workshops, and a resumé. The resumé of each team was then made available to the Congress on the last day. All the conferences given at the symposia, and all resumés, were published just four months after the Congress in a book entitled *Immunology 80*.

The 5th International Congress was organized by the Japanese Society of Immunologists and the IUIS and took place in Kyoto, Japan, on 21–27 August 1983, and was attended by several thousand immunologists. It consisted of 23 symposia and 131 workshops. Amongst the topics discussed were: T-cell activation by antigen, B-cell development, macrophage function, autoimmune diseases, tumour immunology, immunodeficiency, herpes virus immunity, reproductive immunology and transplantation.

Such is the efficient state of organization in immunology that the venues for the 6th and 7th International Congresses are already known. They are Toronto in 1986 and Berlin in 1989.

International Convocations on Immunology

The International Convocations on Immunology began in 1968 and are held irregularly — about every two years.

The 7th Convocation was held at Niagara Falls, New York, in July 1980. It consisted of 40 papers and 30 abstracts from poster sessions. The Proceedings were published as *Immunobiology of the major histocompatibility complex* in 1981. The 8th Convocation was held in Amherst in June 1982 and published as *Regulation of the immune response* in 1982.

The 9th Convocation was held at the Ernest Witebsky Center for Immunology, part of the State University of New York at Buffalo. Its theme was 'Antibodies: Protective, Destructive and Regulatory Role'.

Symposia of the IUIS

The main aim of the IUIS symposia is 'to bridge the generation gap and to give young scientists the opportunity to participate at international meetings of limited size'. For each symposium a well-defined topical subject is selected and considered from various aspects. The meetings generally last four to five days, with an audience of between 100 and 200. The proceedings are not published.

The symposia began in 1971 in Yugoslavia with the title of 'Biological Significance of Transplantation'. Since then, and up to 1984, there have been 14 symposia, the last two being entitled 'Regulation of the Immune Response and

Its Modulation by Infection and Malnutrition' (held in Delhi in November 1982) and 'Autoimmunity' (held at Igls, Austria, in March 1984).

Symposia of the Collegium Internationale Allergologicum

The Collegium Internationale Allergologicum conducts (approximately) biennial symposia; the first was held in 1954. The 13th Symposium took place in Konstanz in July 1980. Its proceedings were published in 1981 as 'Cellular Interactions in Allergy' which comprised volume 66 supplement 1 of the journal *International Archives of Allergy and Applied Immunology*.

Congresses of the European Academy of Allergology and Clinical Immunology

Congress XII of this annual series organized by the European Academy of Allergology and Clinical Immunology was held in Rome in September 1983 and organized by the Italian Society of Allergology and Clinical Immunology under the auspices of the WHO. The main topics discussed included IgE, immunological methods, autoimmunity and immunotherapy. The workshops covered wider subjects.

Congress XIII took place in Brussels in May 1984. Its theme was immunological aspects of asthma, occupational allergy and immunomodulation.

The proceedings are usually published by Elsevier Biomedical in their International Congress Series.

Congresses, Symposia and Meetings of the International Association of Biological Standardization

The International Association of Biological Standardization (IABS) organizes three types of scientific meeting. Its International Congresses are held every two years and relate to problems of research, production and control of immunological products in human and animal medicine. Symposia are held on two or more occasions each year and are concerned with single topics such as poliomyelitis vaccination or standardization of rabies vaccines. Finally, meetings of the Committee on Human Diploid Cell Strains review current developments in the use of diploid cells in vaccine manufacture.

The proceedings of Congresses and Symposia are published in the series *Developments in Biological Standardization* by S. Karger.

Meetings of the British Society for Immunology

The British Society for Immunology (BSI) organized two main types of meetings in 1983. First, there were the four Spring meetings: a Clinical Immunology Workshop entitled 'Abnormalities of Polymorph Function and Opsinization', held in March at the East Birmingham Hospital; a meeting on Avian Immunology at the Royal Veterinary College, London, in April; a workshop on IgA, held at the Institute of Cancer, London, in April; and a workshop on Acute Inflammation, held at the Brompton Hospital, London, in April.

Secondly, and more importantly, there was the Autumn Meeting, which extended over three days (9–11 November) and was held at the Barbican, London. The theme of the meeting was the 'Major Histocompatibility Complex'. It included workshops, symposia, poster sessions and business meetings.

Meetings of the Royal Society of Medicine

Of the many meetings the Royal Society organizes every year, the most relevant in terms of immunological content are those organized by the Society's Section of Clinical Immunology and Allergy. In 1983 these included meetings on 'Cyclosporin A', held in November, 'Targeting and Cancer Therapy' (joint meeting with the Society's Section of Oncology), also in November, and 'The Immunology of the Acquired Immune Deficiency Syndrome (AIDS)', in December. The meetings are usually held at the Society's headquarters in London.

Symposia of the Federation of American Societies for Experimental Biology (FASEB)

The annual meetings of FASEB bring together six societies which make up the Federation — one of which is the American Association of Immunologists (AAI). The meetings, which are held in the spring, are composed of multidisciplinary symposia and members from any of the societies may attend. They are generally thematic; thus in 1983 the themes were 'Calcium' (co-ordinated by the American Society for Pharmacology and Experimental Therapeutics), 'Infectious Diseases' (co-ordinated by the AAI) and 'Neuroendocrinology' (co-ordinated by the American Physiological Society). In addition, the individual societies organize separate mini-symposia, slide and poster sessions, and exhibitions. In 1983 the AAI organized 10 mini-symposia, the topics being: tumour immunology, immunoglobulin and lymphocyte receptors, B-lymphocyte development, activation and immunoregulation, T-cell regulation and lymphocyte function, lymphocyte effector function, immediate hypersensitivity, immunogenetics, macrophage and NK cells, inflammation and complement.

Venues of recent meetings include: Atlanta (65th Annual Meeting, 1981); New Orleans (66th Annual Meeting, 1982); and Chicago (67th Annual Meeting, 1983).

The proceedings of the various symposia are published in *Federation Proceedings*.

As recently as 1982, FASEB initiated Summer Research Conferences with the aim of providing scientists with an opportunity to meet informally to discuss a variety of biological topics. The Conferences are held annually at the Vermont Academy, Vermont. Of the 10 topics organized for discussion in 1984, at least five were of interest to immunologists: immunopharmacology, somatic cell genetics, receptors, mononuclear cells and antibody networks, and development and ageing of the immune function.

4.5 OTHER CONFERENCES

The Transplantation Society has been holding biennial congresses since 1966. The IXth International Congress took place in Brighton in 1982. The Society's proceedings are published in its journal *Transplantation Proceedings*, which appears quarterly, and in the biennial *Transplantation Today*.

The first International Symposium on Immunopathology was held in 1959, and subsequent ones have taken place irregularly since then. The VIIIth Symposium was held in 1980, and its proceedings were published by Academic Press in their series *Immunopathology*.

The Annual Congress for Hybridoma Research, which is sponsored by the journal *Hybridoma*, Scherago Associations and Mary Ann Liebert Inc., was first held in 1982. The second was held in Philadelphia (1983), and the third in San Diego (1984).

One of the longest-running series of conferences is organized by the Reticulo-endothelial Society. The Society was founded in 1963, and the 20th National Reticulo-endothelial Society Meeting was held in Portland, Oregon, in 1983.

The ICN–UCLA Symposia on Molecular Biology have been taking place since 1972. Up to six symposia are held every year of which two or three may be of interest to immunologists. In 1984 symposia on the 'Regulation of the Immune System' and 'Acquired Immune Deficiency Syndrome' were held at the Molecular Biology Institute, Los Angeles.

4.6 CONFERENCE PROCEEDINGS (*see* bibliography entries 55–67)

One of the quieter revolutions to have taken place in the biological sciences over the last few years has been the upsurge in the numbers of books published which are either based on, or verbatim records of, conference proceedings. Sometimes it is obvious that a book represents the proceedings of a meeting: the title may indicate the fact. In other cases (and this may be deliberate) there may be very little indication.

It is easy to see the attraction of conference proceedings to publishers: the editors have a fairly simple task of collecting contributors' manuscripts (which will have formed the basis of the papers they gave at the conference in question), editing them, if necessary, and then adding an appropriate introduction. As a consequence there should be little delay in their publication, particularly in view of modern rapid printing methods; indeed the proceedings of some of the International Congresses of Immunology have been published within four months of the conference. However such speed is rare, and most proceedings take between one and three years to reach publication.

What then are the attractions of proceedings to the readers? Obviously they provide a record of an event that delegates may wish to remember — but except for the International Congresses, the delegates themselves can only represent a very limited audience. Proceedings may bring together information on one topic that may be scattered in the journal and review literature — but with easy photocopying facilities most research workers have little problem in this respect. Finally they may provide original information which cannot be found elsewhere — this is unusual; in most cases papers read at conferences are not new; where they are new the papers are generally on the verge of publication in the journals.

Further drawbacks to published proceedings include the fact that they contain numerous and varying styles; that they are of little use in teaching because their coverage of the topic is uneven and haphazard; and finally that they are expensive.

It is for these very reasons that many conference proceedings are often disguised as something different.

It has been mentioned already that some journals, notably *Federation Proceedings* and *Transplantation Proceedings,* carry the published proceedings of conferences. There are also a number of hardback serials which perform the same function but less frequently.

Elsevier Biomedical are specialists in the publication of proceedings. They have a number of loosely based series which include the proceedings of immunology meetings. Their most extensive series is entitled 'International Congress Series', and today numbers over 600 proceedings. Recent immunology texts in this series include: *Transplantation and clinical immunology,* volume IX (Proceedings of the 9th International Course, Lyon, 1977) published in 1982 (No. 423) and *Fetal liver transplantation* (Proceedings of the 1st International Symposium, Pesaro, Italy, 1979) published in 1980 (No. 514).

Developments in Immunology contains, almost exclusively, the proceedings of various immunology conferences: volume 14 is entitled *Clinical immunology and allergology* (1981) and represents the proceedings of the XIth Congress of the European Academy of Allergology and Clinical Immunology, 1980; and volume 16, *Oral immunogenetics and tissue transplantation* (1982), is the record of an International Symposium held at the University of California, Los Angeles in 1981. *Symposia Fondation Merieux* is mainly concerned with the proceedings of the annual International Courses in Transplantation and Clinical Immunology which take place at Lyon; proceedings of the 13th Course, held in 1981, may be found in volume 7 (1982). *Symposia of the Giovanni Lorenzini Foundation* and *INSERM Symposia* are also sources of proceedings of European conferences published by Elsevier Biomedical.

The International Congresses of Immunology (so far there have been five) have all been published by Academic Press in their *Progress in Immunology* series — volumes I to V; some of them within four months of the meetings.

Immunopathology represents the proceedings of the International Symposia on Immunopathology which began in 1959. One of the most recent is entitled *Immunopathology: VIII International Symposium 1980* and was published by Grune & Stratton in 1982.

Developments in Biological Standardization, a combination of two series, *Progress in Immunobiological Standardization* and *Symposia Series in Immunobiological Standardization,* contains the proceedings of international congresses and symposia held by the International Association of Biological Standardization; volume 52 was entitled *Herpesvirus of man and animal: standardization of immunological procedures* (1982).

The proceedings of ICN–UCLA Symposia on Molecular Biology often contain rich pickings for immunologists; two recent volumes include *Regulation of the immune response* (1984) and *Acquired immuno deficiency disease* (1984).

The International Convocations on Immunology are usually published by Karger, but not as a series; *Immunobiology of the major histocompatibility complex* (1981) and *Regulation of the immune response* (1983) represent the proceedings of the 7th and 8th meetings, respectively.

Three further series which are based on symposia are *Menarini Series on Immunopathology, Perspectives in Immunology* and *Transplantation Today.*

5 Immunology: its literature

5.1 JOURNALS

Introduction

The term 'periodical' is assigned to publications that appear regularly, and usually more frequently than annually. Newsletters, magazines and bulletins are specialist forms of periodical. In science the term 'journal' (in other fields regarded as a synonym for periodical) is reserved for those scholarly/academic publications that carry research papers. Most immunology periodicals are of this kind. Unlike books (and this is their strength), periodicals provide a continuing stream of information which enables them to react and report quickly on current events, issues or research.

Because information in science is such a perishable commodity, and up-to-the-minute information so highly prized, it is not surprising that the periodical has a virtual monopoly in the dissemination of research information. Indeed the demand for current information is so great that publishers are turning to more rapid forms of publishing such as the electronic journal and the unrefereed letter/brief communications journal.

The mainstay of the journal — the ubiquitous article or scientific paper — owes its success to today's need for information packaged in a concise, familiar, and quickly and easily digested form. Constraints on scientists' reading time, and the sheer size of the literature to be assimilated, insist this be the case.

While the article is the most prominent feature of most scientific journals, information of other kinds is also carried. Indeed some journals, such as *Immunology Today*, contain — apart from articles and brief communications — calendars of meetings, job advertisements, book reviews, and professional and product news.

Tracing and locating serials and journals
(*see* bibliography entries 68–93)

Unfortunately, in the library world there is little agreement about the definition and scope of the term 'serial'. This would be of purely academic interest to the immunologist were it not for the sheer size of the population (there were estimated to be 20 000 biomedical serials alone, published in 1977) and the fact that shades of difference in definition can result in the exclusion (or inclusion) of hundreds, if not thousands, of journals from a bibliography or database. So the small print in the preface, when provided, always merits attention. The problem really comes to a head in the coverage (or otherwise) of government publications, newsletters and serial reports. Given then: (a) the uncertainty that surrounds the coverage policies of serial lists; and (b) the variant practices pursued by them, it is probably best, when the choice presents itself, to search sources that do not discriminate between different forms of serial publication. *Conser Microfiche, Keyword Index to Serial Titles* (again in fiche) and the *Index to NLM Serial Titles* are examples of such lists.

There are a rather disconcertingly large number of sources (a conservative estimate would suggest 20) of data on periodicals (the large size of the potential pool of sources is in part a function of the field's interdisciplinarity). The best ones to consult vary according to the nature of the enquiry, and of course on the general availability of the sources. Thus if the title of the journal is known and it is a question of trying to borrow, or browse through it, then we look at union lists (i.e. *New Serial Titles*) or individual library holdings lists (*Periodicals Held by the Science Reference Library*). If on the other hand it is to purchase or verify a title we look through the trade catalogues (e.g. Academic Press's journal catalogue), where price, address and content details are provided.

If the search is being conducted on a subject rather than a title, then obviously only those tools that provide subject search pathways and/or a subject framework are of any value. While *KIST* only caters for a limited 'title-word' subject approach, *Ulrich's International Periodical Directory*, particularly when accessed on-line, caters for both general and specific subject enquiries. In this context the 'journals covered' lists of the major abstracting/indexing tools (like *Index Medicus*) are useful for they offer a unique approach to the titles of other disciplines that regularly carry immunological papers.

For the not too demanding, occasional user, a combination of *Ulrich* and the *Index to NLM Serial Titles* would probably meet most needs. Because of the dynamic nature of the serial literature a once-and-for-all bibliographic description of a serial is really not feasible, and any statement of the serial population is virtually out of date the moment it is published. This is particularly true in a field that is growing as rapidly, and changing as quickly, as immunology. For instance, any list published before 1979 would record less than half of today's population. As a consequence the traditional hard-copy bibliography, with its ponderous publication procedures, is rapidly becoming obsolete and its place being taken by computer-held, or computer-produced, lists which can be updated quickly, easily and cheaply. Examples of such computer-produced lists abound and include *Conser fiche, London University Union List of Serials, Health Sciences Serials* and on-line *Ulrich*.

Comprehensive lists that include immunology

Probably the most heavily used and widely available list of currently published serials is *Ulrich's International Periodical Directory*. It is an annual classified listing, equipped with a title index, that provides all the bibliographic details necessary to enable a periodical to be traced or bought. An attempt is also made, in a rather abbreviated way, to provide some indication of a periodical's contents (i.e. whether it contains reviews, bibliographies, statistics). Also of value are the notes indicating whether copying is free, or photocopies of articles provided. Fortunately immunological journals obtain their own place in the classification scheme, under the heading 'Medical sciences — allergology and immunology'.

Here are listed 62 journals from around the world, although the majority are American. Additionally, references are made to another 11 journals that, because of their multidisciplinarity, have been lodged under other subject headings. Even so, many journals from other disciplines, which do have a significant immunological content, do not merit references. Examples are the *Journal of Experimental Medicine* and the *Journal of Infectious Diseases*.

While *Ulrich's International Periodical Directory* lists only those publications appearing more regularly than annually, its companion publication *Irregular Serials and Annuals*, a biennial publication with an identical format, picks up the annuals, yearbooks, reviews and irregular reports. Under the immunology heading 19 publications are listed. The most effective and speedy way of retrieving data from the two Ulrich publications is to access them on-line, either via DIALOG or BRS. Doing it this way we can search both volumes simultaneously, but more importantly, we can partly overcome the rigidity of the classification scheme by searching all records for, say, the presence of the root *immun*, thus retrieving any publication that has immunology, immunological, immunopharmacology, immunopathology, etc. in its title. This way we would pick up some of those multidisciplinary journals lodged elsewhere. Furthermore we would not lose any of the journals like *Ligand Review*, which do not have the root *immun* in their title, because our search would have also picked up the word immunology as a descriptor. The result of searching with this root is the retrieval of 160 publications, almost double the number that could be identified by the conventional manual search. Most usefully, the on-line version would enable us to identify immediately say US immunological publications, whereas to do so manually would be very laborious because titles in the Immunology section are filed strictly alphabetically, the publications of all countries being inter-filed. The advantages of on-line access do not end here, for to keep abreast of the many changes in the literature in between hard-copy volumes, it would be necessary to consult yet another publication: *Ulrich's Quarterly* (not widely available), which is identical in format to its parent volumes. The on-line file updates itself automatically each month and therefore offers a very current list — and there is still only one place you need to look. The on-line version (but not the manual one) of *Ulrich* also records some dead serials — noting those that have died since 1977.

The on-line *Ulrich* also enables searching under a journal's earlier title and locating it under its new one — an approach rarely catered for in the hard-copy volume, and given the high turnover of journal titles in the field, a very important one. Thus *Transplantation Reviews*, which changed title to *Immunological Reviews* in 1981 (and thus is known by its earlier name to a lot of people), could not be located through the hard copy.

Ulrich offers good coverage of the UK scientific literature; however a useful way of supplementing, and certainly updating, its coverage is through the weekly *British National Bibliography* (*BNB*) which, while avowedly a book bibliography, does in fact list serials and first issues of periodicals. Its subject format makes it possible to mount a search for new immunology titles without knowing their names. Unfortunately the arrangement adopted — Dewey — does scatter immunological publications, so a range of numbers needs examining — 574.29 (general immunology), 591.29 (animal immunology), 581.29 (plant immunology), 616.089 (medical immunology) and 636.089 (veterinary immunology). Accessing *BNB* on-line via BLAISE is perhaps more effective, for here it is possible to retrieve all periodicals with the précis word (pw) *immunology* in their indexing string. Thus *immunology* (pw) and *per* (the code for periodicals) will retrieve all immunology periodicals, and *immunology* (pw) and the code *ser* will retrieve all immunological serials. Such a search on the UKCMARC file (BNB 1977–1983) retrieves, respectively, 15 and 11 titles.

The International Serials Data System (ISDS) is a Unesco organization whose aim is to provide a reliable registry of world serials. The ISDS has sole responsibility for assigning the International Standard Serial Number. A by-product of the ISDS's work is an invaluable bibliographic tool, the *ISDS Register*, which contains approximately 200 000 serials published since 1971. Approximately 30 000 records are added annually to the *Register*. Available annually on microfiche, each *Register* provides a record of the total serials database to that date. The *Register* is updated by the bimonthly *ISDS Bulletin*, which, thanks to a rolling cumulation programme, offers one-place reference. Only an ISSN number and title approach are catered for in both publications; however, these publications are most valuable for their international coverage.

Locating/borrowing serials in the UK

If it is a question of borrowing a particular issue of a periodical, obtaining a photocopy of an article, or obtaining an obscure annual report, then the appropriate tool — certainly in the UK — is *Current Serials Received*, which lists alphabetically by title the 56 000 serials the British Library Lending Division (BLLD) currently receives. This modestly priced publication only provides enough detail to enable a journal to be traced (title and shelf location mark) and its irregular publication (latest edition May 1982) means it can never be truly up-to-date. Those simply seeking the titles of immunology journals, when no names are known, should use another BLLD publication — *Keyword Index to Serial Titles (KIST)*. *KIST* is an alphabetical list of all significant words in the titles of serials; beside each word all the titles containing that word are listed (the system by which titles are ordered and presented is known as keyword-out-of-context). The chances of locating a title are increased by the fact that each journal may be listed in a number of different places (the precise number depending on the number of significant words in its title) and a journal may still be located if the precise form of the title is not known (this is very likely in immunology where so many titles have confusingly similar names). *KIST* is not just a subject guide to BLLD's current serials, for it also covers dead ones as well, and, additionally, it lists the entire serial stock of the Science Reference Library. Well over 200 000 titles, from all countries, are recorded on this fiche index, of which several hundred are immunological in content. Plans are being considered to include the holdings of several other major libraries — Cambridge University, and the Department of Printed Books of the British Library Reference Division (the 'old' British Museum) are mentioned — so what is already an important bibliographic tool could turn into an indispensable means of accessing the major serial resources of the UK.

The *University of London's Union List of Serials*, a relative newcomer to the field (started autumn 1976), is a fiche record of the holdings of the University's 50 libraries. It furnishes 80 000 unique titles including reports, government publications, discussion papers and dead serials. A fairly detailed bibliographic entry (including frequency, classification and location number) is provided in this twice-yearly cumulative publication (there is just one look-up point). The *List* is particularly attractive to the immunologist because it contains the holdings of the universities' 11 medical schools, as well as such important collections as those of the Royal Veterinary College and the London School of Hygiene and Tropical Medicine. Access is of course limited to title, so its value is limited to locating, in London, runs of a specific title for browsing purposes. It is also possible to obtain the *List* in magnetic tape form.

Another British reference work that shows the whereabouts of serials — this time on a national scale — is the recently ceased *British Union Catalogue of Periodicals (BUCOP)*, which incorporated the *World List of Scientific Periodicals*. Its lack of cumulation, the fact that only titles acquired before 1980 are listed, and its title-only arrangement circumscribe its use, but it is invaluable to anyone who wants to browse through journal back numbers, or consult long-established or long-dead titles. Furthermore, a study published in *Interlending Review* (1981) showed that it contained many unique titles not listed elsewhere — around half of the scientific serials listed for instance were not held by the British Library Lending Division or listed in *KIST*.

BUCOP's place has largely been taken by *Serials in the British Library*, a quarterly list of journals acquired by the British Library, and a few specialist libraries. This list gives much more detail for each serial than *BUCOP* ever supplied, though its use also is circumscribed by its alphabetical title arrangement. Cumulations are produced annually on fiche, and confusingly these cumulations contain some titles not listed in the quarterly publications.

Locating/borrowing serials in North America

New Serial Titles lists the serial holdings of over 800 North American libraries. Publications of all countries are included (it is much more comprehensive in this respect than *Ulrich*), with US serials accounting for about a third of the titles listed. Up until 1981 only certain categories of serials published after 1950 were entered; since then however there have been no limitations regarding the beginning date of the publication, or the type of serial admitted. This bibliography is particularly strong in its coverage of newsletters and reports of government, academic and research agencies. Most importantly for the immunologist, *New Serial Titles* is available in both alphabetical title and subject forms. In its subject form it is called *New Serial Titles — Classed Subject Arrangements*. Titles are arranged by Dewey Decimal Classification — a scheme which unfortunately scatters immunological serials, placing the medical ones at 616 (the disease classification number), the zoological ones at 590, the biological ones at 580 and the botanical ones at 579. As immunological serials do not neatly divide up into these categories there is of course some confusion in location. Both title and subject forms of the bibliography are issued monthly, so up-to-date intelligence of the latest holdings is provided. However the real difficulty with using this valuable tool is that it is beset with cumulation problems. Thus a main cumulation covers the period 1950–70 (the title-arranged edition exists in fiche also for this period); for 1971–75 and 1976–79, title-arranged cumulations are available, but not subject ones, and for 1980 to date one has to search annual volumes. It needs no stressing that a search for a journal for which the publication date is not known — surely a common occurrence — can be long and laborious. A subject search could plainly be nightmarish. *New Serial Titles* has, since 1981, been produced by the Conser Project (*Conversion of Serials*); the change has largely been marked by the provision of a full and very informative bibliographic entry.

Table 5.1   OCLC entry for Clinical Reviews in Allergy*

Library of Congress Card Number	84–7088
Cataloguing Source	National Library of Medicine
International Standard Serial Number	0731–8235
CODEN Designation	CRVADD
Authentication Center	National Serials Data Program
National Library of Medicine Call Number	W1 CL 779LF
National Library of Medicine Catline Citation Number	8 30 8524
National Library of Medicine Serial Control Number	C 269 10300
Local Holdings	PNLL
Abbreviated Title	Clin. Rev. Allergy
Key Title	Clinical Reviews in Allergy
Title Statement	Clinical Reviews in Allergy
Imprint	New York, NY: Elsevier Biomedical, 1983–
Subscription Address	Elsevier/North-Holland Science Publishers, 52 Vanderbilt Ave., New York, NY 10017
Physical Description	Printed Serial, Illustrated
Current Frequency	Four Issues
Subscription Price	$80 Institutions; $40 Individuals
Chronological Designation	Vol 1, No. 1 (Mar — 1983–)
Library of Congress Subject Heading	Allergy and Immunology, Periodicals
Holdings	Various
Issue Which Bibliographic Description Based Upon	June 1983

*Only the main fields of description are shown.

The OCLC database, to which the output of the Conser Project is fed, offers what is arguably the most comprehensive locations listing of serials held by North American libraries. An astonishing 600 000 serials or so are furnished with 4 250 000 locations. The right subject flavour of the database is guaranteed by the inclusion of the serial holdings of all the major agricultural, biological and medical libraries, including the National Library of Medicine. Used primarily as an interlending tool in the USA, the database also has an important bibliographic searching function, particularly since it offers what is probably the most detailed bibliographic records of all; it is so expansive that it requires two screens to display it (*see Table 5.1*). As well as the standard bibliographic details, language(s) of contents, classification number(s) and index holding(s) (many of the immunology serials obtain National Library of Medicine classification marks and index headings), previous title and price are also provided.

No subject approach is catered for, nor is any browsing permitted, so its use is very much limited to that of a check-list. Searching is conducted in coded forms, called 'keys', of the serial's title. Initially such searching looks complex and likely to confuse, but it is easily learnt.

A relative newcomer to the field of serial listing is another product of the Conser programme, the National Library of Canada publication (distributed in the USA by the Library of Congress) *Conser Microfiche*. In addition to the listing of the National Library of Canada's serial holdings, it also lists the holdings of 19 other North American libraries, the most important of which is the Library of Congress. It is a three-part publication with a base register 1975–78, annual supplements (both in accession number order) and a cumulative index offering one-place reference to the entire file. It is limited in that it offers only a limited time span of entries, and perhaps more importantly (given the relative recency of the immunological literature), it offers no subject access point — though a search for an organization is possible. Over 250 000 titles are listed in some detail on the fiche (its size is its obvious attraction). As a rough example of its immunological content, two dozen titles were found beginning with the root *immun*. *Conser Microfiche* is also available on magnetic tape.

Subject lists

There are a number of general 'subject' lists though they offer generally less in terms of currency and detail than the comprehensive ones we have previously discussed. In most cases they will not be as immediately accessible either. *Periodicals relevant in microbiology and immunology* promises much from the title, but having last appeared in 1968 it really is of historical interest only. Published by the International Association of Microbiological Societies, it lists around 700 periodicals from 85 countries. Of more value is *Medical serials and books in print*. This handy reference compilation offers, under one cover, subject access to both books and serials. The subject headings are the same as the ones used in *Ulrich's International Periodical Directory* (i.e. serials of interest are listed under the heading 'Immunology' and 'Allergy'); indeed, this is a spin-off publication from the *Ulrich* database so the coverage is also identical.

Of some value are the lists of journals scanned by the major abstracting and indexing services in the field, though they are usually very long and general in character (they embrace either the whole of medicine or biology), lack a subject approach (meaning that the seeker of immunological journals has a long laborious hunt trying to spot a relevant title from the massed alphabetic ranks of medical/biological serials) and offer little bibliographic detail other than title (their function is limited to that of a checklist). *Serials Sources for the BIOSIS Database, List of Journals Indexed in Index Medicus*, its companion publication *List of Serials and Monographs Indexed for Online Users* and the *IRL Life Sciences Collection: List of Journals Abstracted*, are the most important publications of their kind. *Serial Sources* is an alphabetic listing of all journals, review annuals and reports monitored now and in the past by BIOSIS to produce its printed and machine-readable products. Over 9500 currently published serials are listed, as well as over 5000 cessations and titles that have undergone title changes. *Serial Sources* is unusual in that it provides a fairly detailed bibliographic entry (frequency and publishers' addresses are included, for instance). The National Library of Medicine's *List of Journals Indexed in Index Medicus* deserves special mention because it is unusual as it caters for both a subject and geographical approach. Under the subject headings — not keywords — 'Immunology' and 'Hypersensitivity' relevant journals (without bibliographical detail unfortunately) may be found. Altogether nearly 2700 journals are listed.

Another form of 'subject' list is the serial holdings lists of major libraries in the field. Most do publish such lists, although these vary in format from flimsy typescript publications to the bound book for sale bibliographies of such major institutions as the National Library of Medicine. Their value is of course that they provide locations for serials. Additionally, librarians find them particularly useful, as the lists of related libraries offer a useful check against the coverage of their own serial collections.

There are a large number of useful holdings lists published, of which only a selection will be mentioned here (other titles may be located in the bibliography). *List bio-med: biomedical serials in Scandinavian libraries'* subject and geographical scope is self-explanatory. The 1977 published volume and the two supplements (1978 and 1979) list many immunology serials. The National Library's irregularly published *Index of NLM Serial Titles* is probably the most comprehensive and sophisticated of library holdings lists, offering as it does keyword access (36 000 entries in all) to over 5000 biomedical serials. Immunology serials are found under the subject heading 'Immunology' — here 50 are listed. Related titles may be found under the term 'Hypersensitivity'. The *Index* also provides for a search by country, and by an abbreviated form of the journal titles; ceased serials are also listed. The *Index*, designed primarily to meet the needs of users wishing to request serial inter-library loans from the National Library of Medicine, is a product of *SERLINE*, the on-line database maintained by the NLM. *Health Sciences Serials*, a quarterly publication (microfiche only) arising out of the same database, is a useful accompaniment to the above, both in updating it and extending its coverage (it provides location information for 6700 titles held in medical libraries throughout the States). *Health Sciences Serials* is an excellent check-list and inexpensive too. The annually published *Canadian Locations of Journals Indexed for Medline* is a hybrid, offering national locations for the 3000 titles covered by this important indexing service. Only minimum bibliographic details are provided. This locations list forms a sub-set of the *Union List of Scientific Serials in Canadian Libraries*.

Tracing and locating journal articles

There are a rich variety of services whose sole aim, virtually, is to list and report on the publication of journal articles. Something like 90% of all recorded information in science is disseminated in article form, so it is perhaps not so surprising that so many bibliographic services owe their existence to just one form of communication. First, and most important, are the abstracting and indexing services; secondly, the relatively new current-awareness services; thirdly the reviewing services, which are largely selective in their listing and probably the most palatable of them all — immunologists tend to read them as they would any other scientific journal, for primary rather than secondary information; and finally the subject bibliographies which, unlike the others, are normally 'one-off' publications and are universally the products of computer searches — which is why they are discussed in the context of the databases mentioned here.

Abstracting and indexing services

While it is perfectly possible to judge a book by looking at its cover the same certainly cannot be said of journals. The journal itself, in science anyway, is really only a means of transporting information, which is largely packaged in the form of articles. It is mainly because these articles lie buried somewhat anonymously between the journal's covers, that abstracting and indexing journals have arisen; they provide the invaluable service of making an article's publication much more visible. They do this by: providing a variety of search pathways to articles and papers (author, title, subject); drawing together articles published in different journals but on the same topic; and in the case of abstracting journals, summarizing their contents.

Abstracting and indexing journals are current-awareness tools in the sense that they alert users to new articles that might be of interest. Because they must adopt some form of classified arrangement they serve as a broad guide to new developments in the field. Many see it as a particularly important function to trawl widely in pursuit of articles unlikely otherwise to be seen by their readership. *Immunology Abstracts*, for instance, sees itself as a solution to the problem of scatter, which is so endemic in interdisciplinary fields such as immunology; that is, it provides a structure and coherence that are otherwise missing from the literature.

In science some abstracting and indexing services have become so good at their job that they virtually offer the prospect of locating any and every article that has been published in the field since the service's inception. This certainly is the case with *Excerpta Medica* and *Biology Abstracts*. Unfortunately the end-product of such diligence is vast numbers of references, many of dubious worth, which, ironically, in themselves constitute an information problem too big for most to cope with.

Another problem encountered is likely to be the speed with which abstracting and indexing services report on an article's publication: there is inevitably a time lag of some months. In the case of *Immunology Abstracts* this varies between four and six months. Now this gap in listing can be quite crucial, for by definition the most current data are likely to be most useful and the least likely to have been encountered. To fill this gap, publishers have resorted to current-contents lists and more rudimentary forms of indexing (i.e. rotating the words in a journal article's title) and putting the full text of journals on-line as they are published.

With all large and complex abstracting and indexing journals it is easier, quicker and more efficient to search them via their computerized equivalents. This is especially the case when a retrospective search is being conducted. If one is looking for a needle in a haystack — and one often has that feeling when searching through a service that is generating over 100 000 references per year (about par for abstracting journals in science) and has reached over 5 000 000 records in size like *Scisearch* — it is obviously better to do it with the aid of a computer.

Immunology sits rather uneasily astride the fields of biology and medicine and as a consequence it is to both fields that we must look for information on both past and newly published research papers. Both fields have strong, flourishing and well established documentation systems, employing the full range of modern sophisticated retrieval aids (computers being the most notable of these). In theory you should always find what you want, but in practice the very size, sophistication and expense of the documentary apparatus means that it is really only fully employed by the information scientists and the persevering users. The bibliographic apparatus of medicine is probably the most daunting of all. There are unquestionably more — and a wider range of — information tools in the field of medicine than in any other field of scientific endeavour, and there are probably more tools in medicine than in the whole of the social sciences put together. Aslib in their publication *Medical Databases 1983* list 54 computerized services in all, though admittedly some cater rather more for the biological field.

Immunologists are lucky in being served by two excellent abstracting services devoted solely to their needs: *Immunology Abstracts* and *Excerpta Medica* Section 26. Both can be accessed on-line. These two services between them will more than meet immunologists' needs for information on scientific papers. For those with very demanding or specialist needs *Index Medicus, Biological Abstracts* and associated publications, *Science Citation Index, Telegen, Index Veterinarius, Veterinary Bulletin, Abstracts of Microbiology and Hygiene, Biotechnology, Cancerlit, Cancernet, International Pharmaceutical Abstracts* and *Current Awareness in the Biological Sciences* might have to be consulted.

Biological Abstracts (BIOSIS) and related publications. *Biological Abstracts (BA)* has been the standard source of access to the literature of the biological sciences since its inception in 1926. Today, this semi-monthly publication of the Biosciences Information Services (BIOSIS) provides informative, and sometimes lengthy, abstracts in English of currently published research from the biological and biomedical — mostly journal — literature. Over 9000 serial and non-serial publications are monitored, yielding an astonishing 185 000 items per year; and the number of sources monitored is increasing by 100 a year. The scope of *Biological Abstracts* is truly international with something like 50% of the items originating from Europe and the Middle East, 25% from North America, and 4% from Africa.

Each issue of *Biological Abstracts* contains approximately 300 immunology abstracts of about 250 words long, grouped under the following headings: 'Immunology (immunochemistry)' and 'Immunology, parasitological'. Other abstracts relating to immunology, but not located under the above headings, may be found through the subject index (e.g. Lymphocyte/transformation/human). Alternatively, the concept index may be used, which provides for a broader subject approach with abstract numbers being listed under headings such as 'Immunology — parasitology' and 'Immunology/immunochemistry, bacterial, viral and fungal'. An alternative grouping of abstracts can be found in the biosystematic index where they are listed by the appropriate class, order or family where applicable (e.g. *Potyvirus*). Finally an author index and generic index (of little value) complete the volume.

Biological Abstracts' sister publication, *Biological Abstracts/RRM*, provides for coverage of research reports, reviews, meetings, trade journals and books, items generally neglected by *BA*. The format and index provision of *RRM* are identical to that of *BA*, but it only contains citations. Around 150 000 documents are indexed a year.

Probably most people access these two publications on-line either on DIALOG, Data-Star, Orbit, BRS or ESA-IRS, where they are merged to form one database: *BIOSIS Previews*. Apart from the convenience of searching these two publications simultaneously, the best reason for using *BA/RRM* on-line must surely be the sheer size of the database.

At present the BIOSIS on-line database contains over 4 000 000 references dating back to 1969 (abstracts only provided from 1976). In fact it is so large that it is held on three files on DIALOG (1969–76, 1977–80, 1981–), three files on Orbit (1969–73, 1974–79, 1980–) and two on Data-Star (1970–77, 1978–; just one if you use the ZZ facility). The massive relevance of the on-line file can be gauged by the fact that the 1981–84 file on DIALOG lists 2280 documents as containing the phrase monoclonal antibodies, 1584 containing the word hybridoma, and another 701 containing the word hybridomas. The depth of indexing, and the number of search pathways provided, is evidenced by the fact that the various descriptors, concept codes, etc. frequently account for half of the text of any item printed out. Thus, for instance, an article from *Journal of General Virology* (**64**(11), 1983, 2471–8, 'Characterization of monoclonal antibodies to potato virus y and their use for virus detection') was indexed with 21 descriptors, 17 concept codes and 3 biosystematic codes. It is fairly current, having a weekly updated file (on Orbit) with abstracts appearing 3–4 months after the articles have been published: updates are available on-line about five weeks ahead of the printed volume.

All the immunology journals are covered in some depth by *BIOSIS Previews*: thus, looking at the 1981–84 file on DIALOG, *Immunology Today* features in over 150 abstracts, *Immunology* in over 800 and *Immunopharmacology* in over 100.

BIOSIS Previews remains the single strongest database in the field of the life sciences and as such should be the file of first choice for those searching for biological information.

BIOSIS/CAS Selects is the umbrella title for a series of biweekly current-awareness journals, spawned by the BIOSIS and CA (Chemical Abstracts) Search databases, and covering 14 specific biochemical research topics. Each issue contains around 150 abstracts and content summaries arranged in author order. Four of the series are of direct concern to immunology: *Allergy and Antiallergy, Cancer Immunology, Immunochemical Methods* and *Transplantation*.

BIO Research Today is another offshoot of the BIOSIS database, consisting of a group of monthly current-awareness services covering 14 specific research topics, one of which — *Cancer C — Immunology —* is of direct relevance; many more are of peripheral interest (e.g. *Birth Defects*).

Current Awareness in the Biological Sciences (CABS). CABS (not to be confused with the Commonwealth Agricultural Bureaux — CAB) was formerly known as *International Abstracts of Biological Sciences* and has since undergone a major transformation, not least of which is that it is now an indexing service.

The bibliographic citations to articles from 2500 titles are listed under nine main subject headings, one of which is immunology: others of some interest are biochemistry, cell and developmental biology, genetics and molecular biology, and microbiology. Approximately 1300 immunological citations are listed in each monthly issue, distributed throughout the 47 subheadings of the immunology section, and also under the other major subdivisions mentioned above. The latter are clearly signposted at the end of each immunology subheading under the general heading 'These titles are also relevant'.

The format of the journal is unusual, the title of the paper being on the left of the page and the author and bibliographic reference on the right; it certainly is easy to scan.

CABS is also offered on the Pergamon Infoline on-line service. It is available from 1983, currently contains over 150 000 records, and is updated monthly. It is marketed strongly as an unrivalled current awareness/alerting service, but with only a monthly updating programme it can hardly be that: *BIOSIS* of course is updated weekly.

Economy Bulletins, Express Bulletins and Bioscope. The University of Sheffield Bio-medical Information Service (USBIS) is a prolific publisher of specialist biblio-graphic services. It publishes two main types of service: Express Bulletins, which are generated by computerized search profiles, and Economy Bulletins, which are based on sections of *Index Medicus*. There are 58 monthly Express Bulletins in all, covering various areas of biology. For immunologists there are nine of particular interest: *Immunoassay*; *Immunohistochemistry*; *Leucocytes*; *Lymphocytes*; *Macrophages*; *Monoclonal Antibodies*; *Phagocytes*; *Prostaglandins — Biology*; and *Renal Transplantation and Dialysis*. In the main the Express Bulletins are 6–8 page pamphlets, contain-ing between 50 and 100 abstracts and arranged by subject. Generally abstracts are brief (20–30 words) but those in *Immunoassay* are more substantial. The Bulletins also contain a 'forthcoming events' section listing future courses or conferences in the relevant subject areas.

There are over one hundred monthly Economy Bulletins covering more specialized areas of biology. The most relevant immunological ones are: *Antigen–Antibody Reactions*; *Autoimmune Diseases*; *Complement*; *Hypersensitivity*; *Killer Cells and Cytotoxicity*; *Lymphoreticular System and Disease*; *Neoplasm Immunology and Transplan-tation Immunology*. Many more may be of some interest. From January 1984 USBIS began publication of a monthly service called *Bioscope*, which integrates the Express and Economy Bulletins. It comes in five sections, which may be bought separately or together. Section 4 — Immunobiology and Haematology, contains most of the Bulletins mentioned above. *Monoclonal Antibodies*, however, is found in section 5 — Biotechnology.

Excerpta Medica (Embase). The largest, and one of the longest-running, English-language abstracting services covering biomedicine, and consequently demands the attention of the immunologist. Started in 1946, *Excerpta Medica (EM)* now regularly covers 250 000 journal articles (which account for 95% of all entries), conference proceedings, books and dissertations a year. *Excerpta Medica* is in fact not one publication but a series of 44 separate speciality abstracting journals, and two drug literature indexes. The subjects of these publications are geared to the medical specialist's interests. *EM* claims through these various services to cover the most significant biomedical research in all fields and in all languages — and to justify this claim it regularly scans over 4000 journals (but not *Immunology Today*).

Section 26, *Immunology, Serology and Transplantation*, is the *EM* service of most relevance to the immunologist, although items of interest may also be found in Section 4, *Microbiology: Bacteriology, Mycology and Parasitology* (vaccination); Section 16, *Cancer* (tumour immunology) Section 30, *Pharmacology and Toxicology* (immuno-suppressants); and Section 31, *Arthritis and Rheumatism*. Section 26 con-tains some 200 abstracts in each monthly issue. These abstracts are arranged by 24 broad subject headings, which are themselves further subdivided. The major subject divisions are as follows: General aspects; Antigens; Antibodies, Immunoglobulins; Antigen-antibody reactions and complexes; Complement; Hypersensitivity mediated by antibodies; Delayed hypersensitivity; Transfer of immunity; Immunocompetence; Lymphoid tissue; Stimulation of immune response; Immunological tolerance; Specific immunosuppression; Non-specific immunosuppression; Immunological reactions *in vitro*; Allo-antigens of body constituents; Tumour immunology; Transplantation; Chimerism; Graft vs host reactions; Drug hypersensitivity; Immune deficiency and dysproteinemia; Auto-immunity; Laboratory techniques; Miscellaneous; Immunity to infections. Each issue contains an author index and subject index (based upon *EM*'s MALIMET thesaurus), which are cumulated at the end of the year.

Many people will access *Excerpta Medica* through its computerized counterpart *Embase,* which is made available on DIALOG (on three files 1974–78, 1979 to date, and in process records) and Data-Star (where it may be searched as one file using the ZZ facility). On DIALOG the database now consists of a truly massive archive of 2 700 000 records, and is updated biweekly. The database has 100 000 records which do not appear in the printed versions so it is worth using *Embase* on these grounds alone. The time span between the appearance of a journal article and its entry on to the database is between two and five months, although abstracts for 680 or so 'core' journals are sometimes available within six weeks.

The variety and richness of the subject search pathways by which the database can be approached is as much a strength of *Embase* as its comprehensiveness. Three subject vocabularies are offered to the searcher: EMCLAS (the 6500 subject headings used to arrange the hard-copy abstracts), useful for general or broad subject enquiries; MALIMET (Master List of Medical Indexing Terms), a thesaurus of over 200 000 preferred terms and over 250 000 synonyms, which provides for specific subject requests; and EMTAGS, which consists of about 200 general terms describing, for instance, type of article, age of test group, kind of experimental animal, and provides data not included in the article, abstract or citation. Since 1979 subject index terms have been weighted so it is possible to confine a search to documents in which the topic is discussed in detail — in practice a very useful facility.

A look at DIALOG's on-line index for 1980–84 clearly demonstrates how valuable a resource *EM* is for immunologists:

Term	Number of documents
Immunology	93 032
Immunology and allergy	5 540
Immunology and microbiology	3 625
Immunology and serology	80 818
Immunology, hypersensitivity, transplantation	7 404

Even the more specific term 'monoclonal' retrieves 1558 documents from just the In Process file on DIALOG!

An article from *Journal of General Virology* (**64**(10), 1983, 2147–56), 'The effect of proteolytic cleavage of La Crosse Virus G1 glycoprotein on antibody neutralization') demonstrates how thorough the indexing is. This item was provided with the following descriptors: La Crosse virus; virus glycoprotein; virus envelope; cell culture; trypsin; plasmin; and virus antibody; the following tags: cell, tissue and micro-organism culture; chemical and serological analysis and Pr; biochemical and chemical procedures; enzymes; non-human; and viruses: the following identifiers (to supplement descriptors): cleavage of Gl; and altered kinetics of neutralization: and the following section (subject) headings: Virology/RNA viruses/Bunyaviridae/Bunyavirus; Biochemistry, genetics/biochemistry/

enzymology; isolation, cultivation/cell, tissue and organ culture/cell and tissue culture; immunology and serology/immunity to infections/immunity to viruses; and antigens/vital antigens. At over $10 000 for the whole set of *EM* it is by no means cheap; however, most people would probably subscribe to one or two sections, or use it on-line on a pay-as-you go basis. (DIALOG's costs are currently $78 per on-line connect hour.)

Immunology Abstracts (Life Sciences Collection).   *Immunology Abstracts* was the field's first abstracting service, and is still today one of only two devoted exclusively to the immunological literature (the other being *Excerpta Medica* Section 26). Certainly, when it comes to print there is much to be said for a publication that covers nothing but immunology; no unfamiliar classifications have to be grappled with as is the case with general services like BIOSIS.

Immunology Abstracts is published monthly by Cambridge Scientific Abstracts, who are responsible for the publication of another 14 biological abstracting services, of which *Biochemistry Abstracts*, *Microbiology Abstracts* and *Virology Abstracts* are of most interest to the immunologist. Each issue contains approximately 1300 two-hundred-word abstracts (a pointer to the sheer size of the immunological literature). The abstracts are grouped under the following major headings which are themselves further subdivided: Molecular immunology and methodology; Immune response; Immunomodulation; Immunity to infection; Tumour immunology; Histocompatibility and transplantation; Reproductive immunology; and Immune disorders. Interestingly *Immunology Abstracts* has been getting smaller over the years with 15 713 items being abstracted in 1978, but only 12 013 in 1981 (and that in the face of a rapidly growing literature). Coverage of the non-journal literature is a particular strength of *Immunology Abstracts* with books, conferences, bibliographies and reports being abstracted.

Immunology Abstracts is offered on-line together with its 14 companion publications, on the *Life Sciences Collection* database on DIALOG. It is possible to confine the search to the *Immunology Abstracts* subfile, or more usefully one can search the whole file, thus picking up immunological-related material appearing in the other subfiles. Over 5000 journals in 28 languages, as well as the non-serial sources already mentioned, are regularly monitored and their contents abstracted. The file is updated monthly and can only be searched back to 1978, which means of course that for retrospective searching *BIOSIS Previews* must be used. *IRL* is less up-to-date than *BIOSIS* with items taking about five weeks longer to appear, three to four months being the norm between publication and appearance on the *Life Sciences Collection* database. As with *BIOSIS*, items generally appear on the database before they appear in print. Each record on the database is comprehensively indexed with terms drawn from its very own thesaurus — commonly 6–8 are used. A broader search is catered for through section heading codes, which are in effect the subheading used to arrange the print publications.

One of the most useful features of the *Life Sciences Collection* (and a facility you don't get in hard copy) is that you can specify the document form you wish to search — there are 24 to choose from. It is also possible to limit a search to a specific language.

Despite *BIOSIS*'s ascendancy in the biosciences and its growth rate, which is twice that of the *Life Sciences Collection*, the *Collection* still offers the immunological searcher a great deal. It covers nearly 1500 journals not covered by *BIOSIS;*

differences in selection criteria mean that even those journals covered by both services will not always have the same articles selected; and because of differences in indexing practice the searcher is offered different (and perhaps more useful) approaches to the data.

Index Medicus (Medline). *Index Medicus* (*IM*) is another publication from the National Library of Medicine. It is similar to *Excerpta Medica* in that both are information retrieval services concentrating on the biomedical, and especially clinical, literature. The major difference between the two is that *EM* is an abstracting service, while the printed *IM* is an indexing service providing nothing more than the article's bibliographic address. (*IM*'s computerized counterpart *Medline* does however include abstracts for some 40% of the articles on the database.) Like both *EM* and *Biological Abstracts*, *IM* is a massive and quite intimidating publication and is best used on-line.

In its printed form *IM* provides a bibliographic listing of references to current articles from approximately 2600 of the world's biomedical journals (not just medical ones as its name might imply) published in 36 languages. Entries are arranged under specific subject headings (full details of these medical subject headings (MESH) may be found in part 2 of January's *Index Medicus*). References relating to lymphokines for example will be found under the headings:

Lymphokines
    Analysis
    Biosynthesis
    Blood
    Diagnostic use
    Immunology
    Metabolism
    Physiology

Each issue contains an author index and a section entitled 'Bibliography of medical reviews', which contains references to articles that are well-documented surveys of recent biomedical literature; references are ordered by subject heading, e.g. T-lymphocytes.

The individual parts of *IM* are superseded yearly by the *Cumulated Index Medicus*.

IM is offered on-line (in which form it is known as *Medline*) by quite a number of hosts: all provide an archive stretching back to 1966 — a massive 4 500 000 million records in all – but the number of files on which it is held varies: on BLAISE-Link it is held on 5 files, on BRS just 1, on Data-Star 3 (also as one using the ZZ facility), and DIALOG on 3 files.

In fact *Medline* corresponds to more than just the printed *Index Medicus*; the products of *Index to Dental Literature* and *International Nursing Index* are also stored on *Medline*. Since 1975 author abstracts have been furnished for around 40% of all documents. It is possible to limit a search to just those records containing an abstract. Over a quarter of a million records from 3000 journals are added per year, of which nearly three-quarters are English-language. *Medline* is essentially an article-based service, though books were covered up to 1981. The file is updated monthly (*see Premed*, below).

A preliminary examination of the on-line MESH thesaurus, with its search guidance, is certainly to be recommended before embarking upon a search. *Table 5.2* shows a particularly relevant part of this *Index* on DIALOG file 1980–83. Note

Table 5.2   Medline's *on-line index*

Items	Index-term	Related terms
62	Immunologic surveillance	2
2 111	Immunologic technics	33
83 795	Immunology	1
	Immunoperoxidase technics	1
	Immunoproteins (non mesh)	55
3 095	Immunosorbent	
550	Immunosorbent technics	5
182	Immunosorbents	3
2 880	Immunosuppression	8

Source: DIALOG FILE 154.

also the productivity of the terms. In fact some terms (i.e. immunological factors) have become so highly posted that retrieval is unacceptably slow or, in some cases, impossible. To overcome this problem, DIALOG has introduced what are called 'cascaded descriptor codes' for those terms.

Premed, provided on-line by BRS and Data-Star, is a related database specifically designed to provide early access to key medical journals and close the information gap between an article's publication and its appearance on *Medline*. References are to articles, letters, editorials, clinical notes, etc. from 125 key medical journals, corresponding to the *Abridged Index Medicus*. The file provides access only to current records, usually from the most recent three to four months, and is updated weekly.

While *Embase* generally offers more references to the immunological searcher than *Medline*, and in tests has proved to have a more effective retrieval language, *Medline* does extend the scope of *Embase* and, costing something like half the price to search on-line, can provide cheaper access to the same data.

Fairly frequently the National Library of Medicine publishes 'individualized bibliographies deemed to be of wide interest' arising from literature searches of the *Medline* database. Several in the immunological field have been produced since they began publication in 1980. One was on *Lymphocyte hybridomas and their products*, which listed 301 citations to the literature published between January 1979 and December 1980. Another on *Malaria immunology*, listing 368 items published between January 1977 and December 1980, was also issued in 1980. These literature searches are available from the NLM without charge.

IRCS Medical Science Database.   Not strictly an abstracting or indexing service, the *IRCS Medical Science Database* is unique in offering the full text of 32 English-language biomedical journals, for depth searching: of particular note for immunologists is the inclusion of *Immunology and Allergy, Surgery and Transplantation* and *Biomedical Technology*. This BRS database offers the ultimate in up-to-date information as on-line availability occurs simultaneously with print publication. Furthermore IRCS journal publication is very fast, averaging four weeks from receipt of the accepted manuscripts, and guaranteeing current research information.

Tables, figures and references are included in the full-text printout. A special BRS occurrence table and HITS full-text print and display features are provided to enhance printing and scanning of lengthy entries. At present the file can be searched back to January 1982. No controlled descriptors are added to the database.

Science Citation Index (Scisearch).   *Science Citation Index,* an interdisciplinary index to the scientific literature, offers a different approach from the others, although one that is not as novel as it first might seem for it capitalizes upon the time-honoured method scientists have used to follow up their interest in a topic; that is, by examining the citations or references at the bottom of an article of interest. Indeed surveys have shown this is by far the most popular way of searching the literature, the idea being of course that if the article is relevant then so too will be the articles the author cites in support of his or her paper.

Science Citation Index (*SCI*) gathers together all the citations appended to articles, letters, editorials or chapters in the journals and books it covers. It covers annually over 5000 documents, of which about 3300 are journals. All the main immunology journals are included. More importantly, because it is an inter-disciplinary publication — its boundaries being prescribed only by what scientists cite — it will pick up immunology articles, etc. whatever the discipline of the journal they are published in, an extremely important point since immunological research is conducted in so many disciplines.

At the very centre of *SCI* (a three-part work) lies the citation index where, as mentioned above, all citations are gathered together in one alphabetic sequence by the cited author. The particular works cited are listed under the name of each author. Appended to each cited publication are the authors (called source authors) who have cited it. The value of such an arrangement is that if you know that a particular paper is central to your work, then you can find other related, more recent papers, by finding out who has cited that paper (the assumption being that the interests of the two papers are similar). Such a method can relate papers in rapidly changing fields much more effectively than the subject classifications adopted by the more conventional abstracting and indexing services, because it is the researchers (i.e. the subject experts) who are making the subject links. Furthermore, in theory anyway, one supposes that citation indicates value, and thus only the best, most worthy, unique, etc. find themselves indexed by *SCI*. Citation indexing therefore provides, in theory, a degree of selectivity not normally associated with abstracting and indexing services. (The sheer bulk of the publication of course appears to argue against this — it is, however, multi-disciplinary.)

The *Source Index,* and the separately published subject approach to it (*Permuterm Subject Index*), provides details of the items from which the citations forming the *Citation Index* were taken. They themselves form additionally a current indexing service, and can be used separately in the same way as other abstracting and indexing services are used. The *Source Index* in reality comprises three indexes, the first a corporate index listing currently published articles by the geographical location and name of the institutions to which the authors of these articles belong. From this index it is quite possible to establish the productivity of the various research establishments in immunology. If the geographical location of the establishment is not known then the second index should be consulted, which lists organizations alphabetically, each organization's name being accompanied by the details necessary to enable it to be located in the geographic index, where full details of publications are provided. Thirdly there is the source index proper: an alphabetical listing of all the authors of papers that citations have been extracted from. Here full bibliographic details are provided to aid in their location. The very abbreviated style of the reference does take some getting used to, as does the dense format adopted by the whole work. In this respect it is certainly not user-friendly and the reader may be well advised to join most of its users in accessing it in its on-line form (it is available on DIALOG).

The *Permuterm Subject Index* provides the necessary, albeit rather crude, subject pathways to the literature. It is an alphabetical listing of pairs of significant words taken from the title of publications listed in the *Source Index*. The success of the subject search is inhibited by the vagaries of the natural language and addition-ally by the fact that immunology documents can be found under dozens of subject headings, immunology, immunological, immune being the most important. These three headings alone yield almost 1900 entries each bimonthly issue, making *SCI* an important source for immunologists, despite the drawbacks of its layout and bulk.

SCI is known on DIALOG, where it is held on three files, as *Scisearch*. In machine-readable form it is available back to 1974, and constitutes a file of over five-and-a-quarter million records. At $165 per on-line connect hour it is one of the most expensive files covering the immunological field.

Perhaps the greatest use made of *SCI* is a rather vain one: researchers scan it to see whether they have been cited and by whom!

Telegen Reporter (Telegenline).　*Telegenline*, produced by EIC/Intelligence, pro-vides on-line access to the burgeoning literature on genetic engineering and biotechnology. This database is offered on-line by DIALOG and ESA-IRS, and extracts data from over 7000 world-wide sources including new stories, reports, patents, laboratory studies, as well as the traditional scientific paper. The file is noted for its coverage of new products, future markets and new applications, and is quite unique in this emphasis on the economic side of biotechnology. Concise abstracts are provided for each item, and the database may be searched back to 1973. It contains much of interest to the immunologist, with, for instance, a search for items on monoclonal antibodies retrieving 304 documents. Items are indexed fairly generously with an average of half a dozen descriptors. Thus an article in *Science* (18 Nov. 1983, 721), 'Monoclonal antibodies reveal the struc-tural basis of antibody diversity', was indexed by the following terms: MCA Anti IgG; Human gene: IgG; Immunoglobulin, human; MCA production; Mutation, somatic. In addition all records are entered into one of 21 subject categories (review classifications) which allow for broad subject retrieval (e.g. 'Business and economics', 'Research on viral genes'). The file is updated monthly, although a separate weekly 'hotline' is available (*Telegen Alert*) by which subscribers can be notified electronically of 'fast-breaking' developments in areas they have previously nominated.

The *Telegen* database now contains over 10 000 items, so it is relatively special-ized in comparison to, for example, *BIOSIS*. It is also rather expensive at $90 per on-line connect hour. *Telegenline* corresponds to the monthly *Telegen Reporter*. It is possible to obtain the full text of articles summarized in *Telegen* either in fiche or hard copy.

Other related abstracting and indexing services

Veterinary science

The Commonwealth Agricultural Bureaux publish two complementary journals of interest: an indexing service called *Index Veterinarius* and an abstracting service called *Veterinary Bulletin*; both are compiled by the Commonwealth Bureau of Animal Health. *Index Veterinarius* contains 40–50 references to the veterinary immunology literature in each monthly issue, classified under such subject keyword headings as 'immune response' and 'immunity to protozoa'. *Veterinary Bulletin* contains abstracts for about half that number of papers each month, most found under the subheading 'immunology'. Both journals have author indexes. These two information services, together with two dozen of CAB's other bibliographic publications, can be searched on-line on the *CAB Abstracts* database. On DIALOG it is possible to search the monthly updated file back to 1972. A search on the total file under the heading 'monoclonal antibodies, immunology' retrieved 43 references, and one on the descriptor 'immunology' provided over 14 000 references. Helpfully, searches can be limited to a particular language, document type (books, reports, etc. are covered) and to animal or plant references.

Microbiology

Zentralblatt für Bakteriologie, Mikrobiologie und Hygiene (Abstracts of Microbiology and Hygiene) Referate Abstracts is a fairly unexpected source of reference to the immunology literature; but the pickings from this essentially English-language service are indeed rich, amounting to about 200 abstracts an issue, arranged conveniently under the heading 'Immunology', which is itself further subdivided. The abstracts themselves, at 2–3 lines, are very brief.

Biotechnology

Biotechnology is a the name of an Orbit database that covers all aspects of biotechnology, including genetic manipulation and pharmaceuticals. Abstracts are made of articles selected from over 1000 journals, proceedings and patents. *Biotechnology* is a new file produced by Derwent Publications, and can only be searched back to June 1982; it is updated monthly. Corresponding to the print *Biotechnology Abstracts*, the file, at $100 per on-line connect hour, is a relatively expensive source of biotechnology data.

Cancer

The sheer volume of interest in the relatively specific field of cancer is demonstrated by the fact that it has its own on-line databases — two in fact, *Cancerlit* and *Cancernet*. *Cancerlit* is offered up on BLAISE-Link and Data-Star on-line services. Over 3500 journals, proceedings, government reports, books and theses are monitored in the production of the database.

This monthly updated file can be searched for some fields back to 1963, and the immunology of cancer is one of its particular strengths. Since 1980 all documents have been indexed by MESH, so searching the file is very similar to searching *Medline*; indeed since 1983 *Cancerlit* has obtained cancer-related references from *Medline*.

Cancernet on Télésystèmes-Questel corresponds to *Bulletin Signalétique: Cancer/ Oncology B5251* and is a French-language service, but with English descriptors provided. Spanning the period 1968 to date, *Cancernet* constitutes a considerable research archive, particularly with regard to cancer immunology.

The International Cancer Research Data Bank (ICRDB) of the US National Cancer Institute, a contributor to *Cancerlit*, also publishes a series of monthly bulletins called *ICRDB Cancergrams*, which contain abstracts of recently published articles. In all there are 65 of these bulletins; five of these deal specifically with immunological topics: *Clinical cancer immunology and therapy, Immunobiology and cancer — antibodies and tumoral immunity, Immunobiology and cancer — functional aspects of cellular immunity, Immunobiology and cancer — the MHC* and *Viral immunology.*

Pharmacy

International Pharmaceutical Abstracts is available in both print and on-line forms (on BRS and DIALOG). It indexes the international primary pharmacy- and drug-related literature, covering 600 journals (60% of them published outside the USA). It is possible to search the database equivalent through to 1970 — around 100 000 records altogether. This monthly service is particularly useful for picking up useful articles in unusual locations. For example, on the file in 1982 was an article entitled 'Targeting of drugs parenterally by use of microspheres' in *Journal of Parenterology Science and Technology* (**36** (Nov.–Dec.), 1982, 242–8) which was concerned with the use of monoclonal antibodies.

It is possible to limit a search on the database to human subjects and English-language articles.

Economics/industry

Immunology is attracting the interest of investors, industry and businessmen, and as such is rapidly gaining itself a large and growing economic literature. *PTS Promt* on DIALOG is one of the most useful databases for gaining access to this literature. *Promt* monitors over 1000 journals, trade publications, newspapers, government reports, and bank and stockbrokers' newsletters for information on markets, new technology, new products and processes, and industrial production. The file is updated weekly so is quite current, with some items appearing within three weeks of publication.

A sample search on the descriptor 'monoclonal antibodies' produced 28 references from such sources as *Chemical Week, European Chemical News, Journal of Commerce* and *SCRIP — World Pharmaceutical News*. Items are typically like this one abstracted from *Chemical Week* (28 March 1984, 28, 30): 'Two biofirms scale up monoclonals for industry'.

Current-awareness publications (*see* bibliography entries
94–119 for indexing, abstracting and current-awareness services)

Keeping up-to-date with what is being currently published is no easy task, as there are hundreds, if not thousands, of journals which are potential sources of relevant information. Most people, if not because of the sheer time involved but because of the difficulties in finding somewhere that takes all the journals, resort to reference tools that are specifically designed to scan and monitor the literature on their behalf. The conventional abstracting and indexing journals were initially founded to fulfil just such a role, but because they cannot process the data sufficiently quickly for some scientists — and those in immunology are particularly demanding (although computerization has helped) — a new breed of publication, the contents listing, has been introduced to trim back some of this delay.

Current Contents, published by the Institute for Scientific Information, is a series of just such publications. The two titles most relevant to immunologists are *Current Contents — Life Sciences*, and *Current Contents — Agriculture, Biology and Environmental Sciences*. Both services are published weekly (to claim to be current a weekly or fortnightly frequency is essential) and both cover more than 1000 journals, although this total is not reached each week because of the variation in the publication patterns of individual journals. At the centre of these two publications are the facsimile copies of the contents pages of the journals covered in that particular issue. In general these contents pages are about two weeks old when they appear in *Current Contents*. An essential part of these publications is their subject and author indexes. There is also an authors address directory, and one for publishers too, so that offprints may be obtained. The full text of the articles covered by *Current Contents* can be obtained through a document supply service called OATS. The appropriateness of each publication to one's own information needs may be judged by scanning the list of journals covered, which is published twice a year. Retrospective searching, which would otherwise be a nightmare, is made somewhat easier by the appearance of a triennially produced cumulated index. The *Life Sciences* edition covers immunology, and provides contents lists for virtually all of the specialist immunology journals. The *Agriculture, Biology and Environmental Science* edition supplements the data contained in the *Life Sciences* edition with its coverage of such journals as *Phytopathology* and *Veterinary Record*.

Current Titles in Immunology, Transplantation and Allergy is a British-based indexing journal which appears twice monthly, and contains approximately 600 references selected from over 800 periodicals. A classified approach is adopted with the following headings being used:

Immunoglobulins

Lymphoreticular system

The immune response

Antigens

Complement

Immunity to infection

Techniques

Tumour immunology

Histocompatibility antigens

Immunosuppression

Organ transplantation

Type I — anaphylactic hypersensitivity

Type II — cytotoxic hypersensitivity

Type III — immune-complex-mediated hypersensitivity

Type IV — cell-mediated hypersensitivity

Immunopharmacology

Autoimmunity

Unclassified hypersensitivity states

Theoretical and general

The journal also has a feature entitled 'Key references', which provides a selected list of papers that represent current highlights in research, or exceptionally useful reviews, each accompanied by a brief indicative abstract.

Current Advances in Immunology is a monthly publication which began in 1984. It is a product of the CABS database (*see also Current Awareness in the Biological Sciences*) and scans more than 3000 primary journals. Most issues contain around 1400 citations classified under 50 major headings. The format is identical to that of *Current Awareness in the Biological Sciences* with title of article on the left and the authors and addresses on the right. At the end of each subject heading there is a list of cross-references. There is an author index.

Finally, the most recent addition is *BioEssays*, a monthly current-awareness journal that also features news and reviews of molecular, cellular and developmental biology, *BioEssays* is co-sponsored by members of the ICSU and its member organization the IUIS.

Immunology journals

Immunology is saturated with journals — a sure sign of considerable research activity. For the researcher newly embarked upon the field, and for the librarian charged with buying them, the choice must be bewildering — and furthermore the choice is ever widening. The prospects for the established researcher, faced with an overburdening reading load, are perhaps not much better. There are now some 80 journals publishing immunological research — and the number is rising fast. To this formidable reading list must be added: (a) the half dozen or so general scientific, medical and veterinary journals (i.e. *Nature*, *The Lancet*) that have traditionally found space for the reporting of significant immunological research, and (b) those journals that concern themselves with the nebulous but related area of molecular biology, journals such as *Molecular and Cellular Biology* and *Cell Biology*. Altogether then there are, at the very least, 150 journals that immunologists might have to concern themselves with at some time or other.

The explosion in the number of immunology journals is best portrayed graphically, as *Figure 5.1*. In little more than a decade (1970–83) the periodical population has tripled in number, and at a time when, because of a downturn in research, library and national budgets, most other fields of knowledge have registered nil or negative growth. Rather disconcertingly for the immunologist, growth shows no signs of abating, and if the rate of growth maintains itself at current levels the periodical population will have increased to well over a hundred, by the end of the 1980s.

The burgeoning literature is of course just one manifestation of the tremendous surge of interest that has been shown in immunology in the academic, medical and business worlds. That interest has mushroomed throughout the biosciences, touching upon such fields as microbiology, molecular biology, biochemistry, pharmacology, cancer, genetics, neurology, pathology, and most recently toxicology — and all of these subjects have boosted the population by giving birth to their own 'immuno' journals (i.e. *Immunogenetics*, *Immunopharmacology*).

Core journals

Because of the seemingly infinite amount of information available to the immunologist, selection is of paramount importance, although selection will, in part, be dictated by availability, access and of course habit.

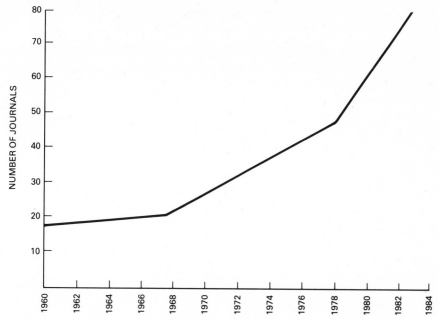

Figure 5.1 Growth in the population of immunology journals, 1960–83. (Only those titles whose primary function is to carry immunological information have been counted)

One method of limiting the journal population to a manageable number without too great a loss of information, is to identify the 'core' journals of the field. It is a well established law of scientific communication that a small percentage (6% is commonly cited) of journals (called 'core' journals) carry something like 90% of the scientific communication in the field. (The percentage is likely to be somewhat higher — possibly 10–12% — for interdisciplinary fields like immunology.)

One way of determining the core journals in the field is to examine a relevant indexing or abstracting service to see which journals are covered most frequently. Being a largely quantitative exercise this naturally favours those journals appearing most frequently and carrying most articles. Such an exercise can provide valuable data to support personal or corporate decision-making: in particular you might consider those journals at the top of the rankings that are not presently being taken, and also those ones at the bottom of the rankings that *are* being taken, and then justify your present purchase patterns (there might, of course, be very good reasons for a departure from the rankings!).

Table 5.3 gives the results of such an exercise based upon an examination of the 1982 volume of *Current Titles in Immunology, Transplantation and Allergy,* which is published twice monthly by MSK Books (London). This service scans some 800 periodicals (an indication itself of the scatter of publication in the field) and indexes some 600 papers per issue. From the table it can be seen that just 20 journals (3% of those that are scanned) account for around 60% of the abstracted papers. What is equally interesting is how evenly relevant information is

Table 5.3 Journals most frequently cited in Current Titles in Immunology, Transplantation and Allergy *(1982)*

Rank	%	Cum.%	
1	8.7	8.7	*Journal of Immunology*
2	4.7	13.4	*Cellular Immunology*
3	4.4	17.8	*Transplantation*
4	4.1	21.9	*Clinical and Experimental Immunology*
5	3.7	25.6	*Journal of Immunological Methods*
6	3.6	29.2	*Proceedings of the National Academy of Sciences*
7	3.1	32.3	*Journal of Experimental Medicine*
8	3.0	35.3	*Infection and Immunity*
9	2.9	38.2	*European Journal of Immunology*
10	2.8	41.0	*Journal of Clinical and Laboratory Immunology*
11	2.6	43.6	*Clinical Immunology and Immunopathology*
12	2.3	45.9	*Immunology*
13	2.0	47.9	*Cancer Research*
14	1.9	49.8	*Tissue Antigens*
15	1.7	51.5	*International Archives of Allergy and Applied Immunology*
16	1.5	53.0	*Scandinavian Journal of Immunology*
=17	1.4	54.4	*Arthritis and Rheumatism*
=17	1.4	55.8	*International Journal of Cancer*
19	1.3	57.1	*Immunopharmacology*

dispersed amongst the leading journals. The obvious exception is *Journal of Immunology*, which accounts solely for almost 10% of the abstracted items. The length of the tail — long tails are characteristic of interdisciplinary fields — is also a feature of the table, meaning many, many, journals annually carry just one, two or three items of interest to immunologists.

A more qualitative approach to establishing the worth of a journal can be made by ranking journals according to the number of citations made to them in review articles appearing in a high-quality review series such as *Advances in Immunology*, the assumption being that only the worthy are cited. This particular series, published by Academic Press, appears annually in two volumes and consists of some 12 topical full-length reviews complete with copious references. *Table 5.4* shows those journals most frequently cited in *Advances in Immunology* in 1981. Once again the *Journal of Immunology* is confirmed as the key journal in the field, accounting now for over a quarter of all citations. Note also that the top 20 journals derived from this method account for over 90%, not 60% as previously shown, of the total citations, indicating perhaps the considerable redundancy in the literature. The fact that 10 of the titles are common to both lists suggests that in such a diffuse field some degree of consensus prevails.

The importance of 'scientific' journals like *Nature* and *Science* is also underlined by this exercise. While the number of immunology papers appearing in them is

Table 5.4   Journals most frequently cited in Advances in Immunology
(1981)

Rank	%	Cum. %	
1	27.0	27.0	*Journal of Immunology*
2	18.0	45.0	*Journal of Experimental Medicine*
3	8.0	53.0	*Nature*
4	6.5	59.5	*Cellular Immunology*
5	6.0	65.5	*European Journal of Immunology*
6	5.0	70.5	*Proceedings of the National Academy of Sciences*
7	3.0	73.5	*Immunology*
8	2.5	76.0	*Science*
=9	2.0	78.0	*Immunological Reviews*
=9	2.0	80.0	*Clinical and Experimental Immunology*
=9	2.0	82.0	*Scandinavian Journal of Immunology*
=12	1.5	83.5	*Journal of Clinical Investigation*
=12	1.5	85.0	*Federation Proceedings*
=12	1.5	86.5	*Transplantation Reviews*
=15	1.0	87.5	*Cell*
=15	1.0	88.5	*Blood*
=15	1.0	89.5	*Experimental Cell Research*
=15	1.0	90.5	*Clinical Immunology and Immunopathology*
=15	1.0	91.5	*Lancet*
=15	1.0	92.5	*Transplantation*

relatively small, those that do are of great significance and are therefore cited frequently.

Though the above two exercises are useful in helping to identify what are generally regarded as the most important journals in the field they do, however, discriminate against the highly specialized journals that are not widely used, but nevertheless contain subject information not usually found elsewhere. Neither do the exercises take into account the relative subject strengths of even the more general journals listed in the tables. To correct for this failing, *Table 5.5* lists those journals that contribute most significantly to the various specialisms found within immunology. The subject headings used in the tables are based on those of *Current Titles in Immunology, Transplantation and Allergy.* The data were obtained from the same source.

Individual immunology journals *(see* bibliography entries 135–230)

On the surface, the various immunology journals look remarkably similar and many have confusingly similar titles, but on closer scrutiny it is possible to discern some differences which enable them to be grouped loosely into five types. First, there are the 'conventional' scientific periodicals containing full-length original

Table 5.5 Journals specializing in the various sub-fields of immunology

Subject	Journal
Immunoglobulins	*European Journal of Immunology; Journal of Immunology; Molecular Immunology; Nature; Proceedings of the National Academy of Sciences (USA); Developmental and Comparative Immunology*
Lymphoreticular system	*Journal of Immunology; Journal of Clinical and Laboratory Immunology; Journal of Experimental Medicine; RES — The Journal of the Reticuloendothelial Society* (since 1984 the *Journal of Leukocyte Biology*)*; Journal of Clinical Investigation*
The immune response	*Journal of Experimental Medicine; Clinical and Experimental Immunology; Cellular Immunology; Clinical Immunology and Immunopathology; European Journal of Immunology; Journal of Immunology; Immunology*
Antigens	*Proceedings of the National Academy of Sciences (USA); Infection and Immunity; Immunological Communications; Vox Sanguis; Molecular Immunology*
Complement	*Journal of Immunology; Complement; Nature; Clinical Immunology and Immunopathology*
Immunity to infection	*Infection and Immunity; Parasite Immunology; American Journal of Veterinary Research; Journal of Clinical and Laboratory Immunology; Journal of Immunology; Journal of Infectious Diseases*
Techniques	*Journal of Immunological Methods; Cancer Research; Clinical Chemistry*
Tumour immunology	*Cancer Research; Cancer Immunology and Immunotherapy; International Journal of Cancer; Cellular Immunology; Cancer Research; Journal of Immunology*
Histocompatibility antigens	*Tissue Antigens; Human Immunology; Journal of Immunology; European Journal of Immunology; Immunogenetics*
Immunosuppression	*Transplantation; Clinical Immunology and Immunopathology*
Organ transplantation	*Transplantation; Clinical Immunology and Immunopathology; Proceedings of the National Academy of Sciences (USA)*

Table 5.5 (continued)

Subject	Journal
Hypersensitivity	*Clinical and Experimental Immunology*; *Allergy*; *Arthritis and Rheumatism*; *Annals of Allergy*; *Clinical Allergy*; *International Archives of Allergy and Applied Immunology*
Immunopharmacology	*Immunopharmacology*; *Molecular and Cellular Biochemistry*; *Cellular Immunology*; *Annals of Allergy*
Autoimmunity	*Arthritis and Rheumatism*; *Journal of Clinical and Laboratory Immunology*; *Cellular Immunology*; *Journal of Immunology*

research papers and very little else. Secondly, there are those whose strength lies in the rapid dissemination of research; they present information in the form of relatively short research communications. A third group concern themselves with reviewing and interpreting the original research of others. Fourthly, there are the 'popular' journals-cum-newsletters which relate news, reviews, announcements and some original research in a 'user-friendly' magazine style. Finally there are a small number that carry the proceedings of meetings, seminars or conferences held by professional societies, or international bodies. There is, however, much overlap between the groups with, for instance, a few conventional scientific journals providing space both for reviews (albeit probably one per issue) and short communications.

One final point to bear in mind is that its title is not always a good guide to a journal's content: some sound all-encompassing but only cover small areas. Others have specialist titles and yet are more comprehensive than one would be led to believe. Concise descriptions of the various journals of direct relevance to immunologists follow. A standard description of each journal is not offered, rather the main strengths and characteristics of each one are emphasized.

Conventional scientific periodicals
Undoubtedly, the premier journal in the field is the long-established *Journal of Immunology*, the official organ of the American Association of Immunologists since 1916. Not only is this popular journal (circulation 8000) the most highly cited periodical in immunology by whatever measuring method one employs, its coverage of immunology is also the widest in scope. The 70 or so papers appearing every month (a sizeable output by any standard) covers work in all areas of immunology, but with some emphasis on the lymphoreticular system, the immune response, cancer and histocompatibility antigens. A number of short communications, announcements of forthcoming meetings, and advertisements complete the journal's contents.

A much more recent publication is Academic Press's *Cellular Immunology*, which has, in a short space of time (it was first published in 1970), become one of the leading journals in the field. Although it has less of an output than the *Journal of Immunology*, it does publish work in much the same areas, with perhaps a little more emphasis on the field of immunopharmacology. Unusually, *Cellular Immunology* reports 18 times a year — a frequency which ensures rapid publication of research findings — and usefully provides a forthcoming list of titles and an author index in each issue.

By its title one would not expect the *Journal of Experimental Medicine* to be a major source of immunological information; in fact its contents are almost exclusively immunological, and its importance in the field is confirmed by the fact that it is the second most heavily cited journal in the 1981 volume of *Advances in Immunology*. This monthly journal is one of the oldest in the field, having been founded in 1896, and as a result of its longevity carried reports of much of the early immunological research. Today the 20 or so long, and five short, communications cover two main subfields: the lymphoreticular system and the immune response. The *European Journal of Immunology*, a West German periodical publishing in English, covers similar ground but additionally publishes work on histocompatibility antigens. It is a monthly journal containing some 15 papers, as well as three to four short articles; it occasionally includes official reports on topics such as nomenclature in immunology.

The leading British journal, established in 1958, some forty years after its US counterpart, is simply entitled *Immunology* and is published monthly by Blackwell Scientific for the British Society for Immunology. The 20 or so papers an issue cover most areas of the subject fairly evenly; methodological papers are however rather rare. Book reviews and advertisements are also a feature of the journal. While it merits the attention of half a dozen abstracting and indexing services, and attracts a circulation of over 2500, *Immunology* has a relatively low rank (7th) in terms of the citations it receives in *Advances in Immunology*. The *Journal of Immunology* by comparison attracts nine times as many citations. *Clinical and Experimental Immunology* is another British Society for Immunology monthly, but differs from *Immunology* in placing more emphasis on the role of immunology in the diagnosis and pathogenesis of disease, particularly in the area of hypersensitivity. Rather more expensive than its sister publication, *Clinical and Experimental Immunology* has a circulation of just under 2000.

Published by Blackwell Scientific on behalf of the Scandinavian Society of Immunology, the monthly *Scandinavian Journal of Immunology* is international in its coverage of immunological research and the latest developments in investigative techniques. It is the practice of the journal to publish supplements on topics deserving lengthy and detailed discussion; this it does frequently, 10 having appeared since 1981. The journal is highly thought of, ranking 10th in the citation exercise, and has a circulation of a little over 1000.

Clinical Immunology and Immunopathology, another Academic Press journal, publishes papers concerning normal and abnormal aspects of immunology, with a particular emphasis on the lymphoreticular system and immune response. The dozen papers appearing monthly may also include two brief communications. The *Journal of Clinical and Laboratory Immunology* is a specialist publication working in the field of the lymphoreticular system; articles on cancer, hypersensitivity and autoimmunity are also published. Easily recognizable by its attractive and colourful front cover, the *International Archives of Allergy and Applied Immunology*, published by S. Karger in Basel, appears to provide for most aspects of immunology, with allergic and related disease featuring strongly. This long-established journal (1950–) appears monthly, and contains about 15 full-length articles, the occasional short paper, and several book reviews. The leading journal in the field of methodology is the *Journal of Immunological Methods*, which ranked fifth in *Current Titles* in 1981. Published fortnightly, it is one of the most frequent journals in the field. About a dozen papers are carried per issue, in addition to book reviews, announcements and immunotherapeutic news. Available only as an integral part of the above journal is a supplement entitled *Monoclonal Antibody Information*, which disseminates information concerning potentially valuable monoclonal antibody-secreting cell lines which investigators are willing to make available to others. The *Journal of Immunoassay*, started in 1980, is a recent recruit to the field; its specialism is enzyme immunoassays and other methods, although it is only published quarterly. The recently introduced (1983) *Journal of Molecular and Cellular Immunology* aims to cover similar areas.

Tissue Antigens, a Danish publication, is a monthly specialist journal which enjoys a relatively large readership; it concentrates mainly on the histocompatibility antigens, as does the quarterly *Human Immunology*, the official journal of the American Association of Clinical Histocompatibility Testing, which has appeared quarterly since its inception in 1980.

Increased research activity in immunogenetics over the last decade has led to the publication of three journals devoted to this field: *Immunogenetics*, *Journal of Immunogenetics* and, most recently, *Experimental and Clinical Immunogenetics*.

Transplantation publishes papers in the field of organ transplantation and related areas such as immunosuppression, histocompatibility antigen. Some papers on the immune response also appear.

Immunopharmacology, the *Journal of Immunopharmacology* and the *International Journal of Immunopharmacology* are three journals, all launched in 1979, servicing this increasingly important subject hybrid of immunology and pharmacology. The first is the most widely abstracted of the three, and also the most frequent, publishing eight times per year.

Until the appearance of the bimonthly *Cancer Immunology and Immunotherapy* in 1976, most of the research in tumour immunology was published in journals such as *Cancer Research* and *International Journal of Cancer*. While these and the ubiquitous *Journal of Immunology* still provide this information, the aforementioned journal is establishing itself as an authority in cancer immunology. It also covers other biological response modifiers.

Parasite Immunology, a specialist publication with a circulation of less than 500, contains papers on host control of parasites — not just helminths and protozoa but also micro-organisms — and the immunopathological reactions that take place as a result. *Infection and Immunity* places greater emphasis on micro-organisms and the 60 or so papers in each issue are divided into the categories Microbial Infections; Viral Infections and Immunity; Oral Microbiology and Immunity; Pathogenic Mechanisms; and Immunology. *Veterinary Immunology and Immunopathology* specializes in the immunology of domestic and laboratory animals, and was first published in 1980.

Quite a number of journals direct themselves solely to the field of allergy/hypersensitivity. Foremost of these are: *Arthritis and Rheumatism*, a monthly periodical published by the Arthritis Foundation of Atlanta, which has, by immunology standards, a large circulation of some 8000; *Clinical Allergy*, published bimonthly on behalf of the British Society for Allergy and Clinical Immunology; *Allergy*, formerly *Acta Allergologica*; and *Annals of Allergy*, published monthly by the American College of Allergists in Minneapolis. *Allergy* also includes selected abstracts from other periodicals in related fields.

Rapid communications

There are six major journals devoted to the rapid dissemination of immunological information; four of these have appeared since 1979. The oldest, *Immunological Communications,* was first published in 1972 and, like the others, is designed to reduce the time lag between submission of a manuscript and its publication. In this case the lag varies from two to three months. It aims to cover all facets of fundamental and applied immunology. This bimonthly journal of the Center for Immunology at the State University of New York contains about seven papers an issue, some book reviews, and announcements. *Immunology Letters* is the official journal of the Federation of European Immunological Societies and is another vehicle for rapid communication of short complete reports in all aspects of immunology. *IRCS Medical Science: Immunology and Allergy* is one of 32 specialist IRCS journals started in 1982 covering the entire field of biomedicine. Each monthly issue contains about 10–11 short communications giving only essential details; these usually amount to papers of 1000 words. The publishers say that publication takes 15–45 days from receipt, whereas by comparison the standard scientific journal might take eight months to a year. In addition to *Immunology and Allergy* some immunology may be found in two other IRCS journals, *Cancer, Surgery and Transplantation* and *Haematology.* Usefully the full text of all papers is available on-line through commercial vendors. The quarterly *Survey of Immunologic Research,* first published in 1982, provides a mixture of guest editorial reviews (five in its second issue), symposium papers and research papers, under the headings 'Hypotheses and Theories', 'Clinical Immunology Reviews' and 'Discussions on Methodology'. The articles are short, rarely exceeding 1000 words. *Thymus,* a bimonthly published by Elsevier from Amsterdam, is a more specialized publication containing short papers within the field of thymology and cellular immunology. *Molecular Immunology,* formerly known as *Immunochemistry,* professes to publish preliminary communications within eight weeks of receipt. It covers those immunology papers that 'can be delineated at the molecular level'. Some reviews and proceedings of meetings are also published.

Interestingly, few of these journals achieve high citation figures and it might well be that they are regarded as rather ephemeral, albeit useful, sources of information, partly perhaps because they are not subjected to the full rigours of the refereeing process and partly because their print style is unattractive.

Review journals

While many journals will include at least one review of an immunological topic per issue there are a number that exclusively deal with reviews. The oldest of them is *Immunological Reviews,* formerly *Transplantation Reviews,* but because of its irregular appearance, about three times a year, it will be discussed under 'Review publications covering immunology'. *CRC Critical Reviews in Immunology* has appeared quarterly since 1980 and carries a couple of topical reviews in each issue on a wide range of immunological subjects. *Clinical Reviews in Allergy,* begun in 1933, publishes a number of review papers devoted to a single topic in each quarterly issue, e.g. 'The mast cell'. *Clinical Immunology Reviews,* a twice-yearly publication, is another recent addition to the review literature.

First published in 1978, the quarterly *Springer Seminars in Immunopathology* provides good, short review articles on immunological subjects with clinical relevance. *Survey of Immunologic Research* contains a high proportion of reviews, as do *Immunology Today*, *Nature*, *Science* and *The Lancet* (*see* the next section).

Popular journals ('mediating' journals)

Immunology Today has done much in its short time of existence to popularize immunology by providing, at relatively low cost, a readable source of information. It contains highly topical review articles, critical commentaries, speculation, news features, book reviews and a very comprehensive diary of forthcoming conferences and courses (in other words it provides a full information service, sufficient to keep its readers abreast of the various 'happenings' in the field). Published separately are a number of teaching aids in the form of charts and diagrams of immunoglobulins, etc. This monthly journal can (and should) be read by undergraduates, teachers, doctors and research immunologists. More for the clinician is the monthly *Clinical Immunology Newsletter*, which began in 1980. This G. K. Hall publication issues original articles of practical interest, on such topics as diagnostic methods and techniques for interpreting laboratory results. Other sections include case reports, questions and answers, and correspondence. Much applied immunology will also be found in *Clinical Chemistry*, which contains original papers, reviews, scientific notes, letters, case reports, history, obituaries, book reviews and announcements. This monthly journal of the American Association for Clinical Chemistry has a circulation in excess of 13 000. It is arguable that the *Journal of Immunological Methods* should also be included here as it contains some news, reviews, announcements and book reviews, in addition to scientific papers.

Unquestionably the most popular, widely read and prestigious journals in the field are the three general scientific weekly magazines — *Nature*, *Science* and *The Lancet*. While other publications may be consulted irregularly, or as the need arises, these magazines are read regularly, with pleasure, as part of a scientist's general current-awareness activity.

Nature is undoubtedly science's most prestigious journal, and also one of its longest-running (it was first published in 1869). It is a multi-format publication, containing opinions, news features, reviews, articles and letters (which are truly short, informative and highly original communications). All the major immunological breakthroughs were first reported in its pages, an example being Kohler and Milstein's monoclonal antibody production. Most of the immunological work published in *Nature* relates to immunoglobulins. *Science*, published by the American Association for Advancement of Science, has been going for even longer than *Nature*, predating it by 20 years. It is much like *Nature* in format, containing articles, news and comment, research news and reports (which like *Nature*'s letters are short and highly original communications). *The Lancet*, one of the oldest scientific journals still extant, publishes both UK and North American editions, and contains news, editorials, surveys, reviews, and some 30 brief original communications. The immunology that is reported here is generally of clinical importance.

Because these three publications figure highly in authors' publishing aspirations the quality of the papers is always of a very high order. This concentration of excellence proves most helpful to those scientists with only limited reading time, especially practitioners. To the scientific researcher who works in a narrow, very focused field, these magazines offer an unusual breadth of vision and, perhaps as a result, encourage important cross-fertilization between fields of scientific activity.

Finally, for those requiring ideas, analysis and information on the biotechnological side of immunology, the authoritative forum is *BioTechnology*, a monthly journal first published in 1983.

Journals carrying proceedings of meetings, etc.

Transplantation Proceedings, the official quarterly publication of the US-based Transplantation Society and the Japanese Society for Transplantation, encompasses the seminars and workshops of these two societies. It also contains reviews and correspondence. Three journals already mentioned, *Survey of Immunologic Research, Molecular Immunology* and *Immunological Communications*, may also devote some space to the inclusion of conference proceedings. *Proceedings of the National Academy of Sciences* (USA) and *Federation Proceedings* also carry the proceedings of conferences where immunology is occasionally a topic.

5.2 REVIEWS AND MONOGRAPHIC SERIES

Scientists do not generally suffer from a shortage of information; indeed most are inundated with it. As a consequence they usually require help not in finding more information but in selecting the most valuable or relevant information from a literature that is said to be doubling in size, at least, every ten or fifteen years. Abstracting or indexing services cannot provide the answer as they really only construct search pathways through the literature. They can do nothing by way of reducing its bulk; indeed, because they have the unfortunate habit of paralleling growth in the primary literature, they actually add to it. Furthermore it has been clear for many years now that the scanning of indexes and abstracts is proving too much for many workers, despite the added convenience of on-line access. Thus a more easily digestible alternative is needed.

What has been seen increasingly as the solution to the information problem is the review. Reviews take the form of a critical summary of current developments in a particular field, and are normally written by eminent specialists; the level of eminence, of course, depending on the prestige of the serial or journal. The philosophy behind the review is a simple and worthy one: from a literature of say a thousand or so research papers, the reviewing author selects perhaps a hundred of the most noteworthy, filtering out as a result the run-of-the-mill and less valuable. The prospect of someone — and an important someone at that — reducing the literature to such manageable proportions is a particularly attractive one to the besieged immunologist, to whom the literature search is only a secondary, possibly tiresome, activity anyway.

The value of a review hinges upon the author's critical powers and, ultimately, the quality of his selection. To make a valid selection in the first place the author must have surveyed the total pool of potentially relevant papers. Now to do this properly requires not only plenty of time but also considerable bibliographic expertise (in first establishing that a relevant paper exists and then locating and obtaining it). In such an interdisciplinary field as immunology, where items may emerge at any time from a number of possible outlets, the task is that much harder.

It must be remembered however that exhaustiveness is not the chief criterion by which a review is judged; nothing is in fact duller and less helpful than those meticulous papers (and immunology has its lion's share) that mention every fact and paper no matter how trivial — a review of 700 or so papers is by no means uncommon. And when one considers that the only form of criticism employed by authors of reviews is omission, then it becomes clear that many so-called reviews are nothing more than annotated bibliographies masquerading as reviews. Adding the fact that personal bias can intrude, one can easily see that the review is not the panacea it was once thought to be.

Reviews may appear in a number of different locations: as articles in journals, chapters in books, papers in conference proceedings, or grouped conveniently together in publications of their very own — the annual review of progress. However, whatever the location, their function, purpose and content are essentially the same. What might differ however is their topicality — the most up-to-date are likely to appear as papers given at conferences, and the least current in textbooks — and complexity — journal reviews are likely to be written at an advanced level.

Review publications covering immunology
(*see* bibliography entries 231–269)

With an overabundance of primary journals in the field it is probably not surprising to learn that there is no shortage of reviews either. Indeed perhaps one would expect numbers to go hand-in-hand if the reviewing system was operating effectively in this rapidly expanding field. The importance of someone standing back and taking regular stock of developments is brought home by the fact that the field has four journals that carry nothing else but reviews: *CRC Critical Reviews in Immunology, Clinical Reviews in Allergy, Clinical Immunology Reviews* and *Springer Seminars in Immunopathology*. (Virology by way of comparison has none.)

However it is the annual or, more commonly, irregular serial that carries the major burden of reviewing research. There are 26 that exclusively cover immunology, and another 20 have some relevance to the field. In the main they are all written for the more general reader, and appeal in particular to students, teachers and researchers working outside their own specialization. They do, of course, also offer a convenient starting point for a retrospective literature search.

These 'serial reviews' — for want of a better name — share a number of characteristics: they are hardback and bear a strong physical resemblance to books, with which they are easily confused; they are published infrequently — either annually, irregularly, or in some cases erratically (hence further confusion with books); they usually contain words such as 'review', 'advances', 'current topics', 'progress', or 'developments' somewhere in their title; and they are all multi-authored.

Monograph series may easily be mistaken for review serials, particularly in the case of the erratically published, one-topic kind. In fact most of these so-called 'series' are nothing more than a loose assemblage of quite disparate books issued under an umbrella title (in an attempt to boost publishers' sales) and display no intention of reviewing published research. In fairness, the lines are not always easily drawn; most books attempt some review of the literature. So in cases where there is likely to be confusion in the user's mind, a monograph series has been listed here and in the chapter on 'books', where reference to all the other monograph series will also be found.

It is almost impossible to assess the relative merits of the various review serials in the field, so what follows here is a general description of all the older-established publications, and some of the newer additions.

The best-known and most authoritative review series is *Advances in Immunology*, which began publication in 1961; it reached volume 35 in 1984. To keep abreast of the rapid developments in immunology over the last few years the publishers are producing two volumes a year. Generally half a dozen fifty-page reviews are contained in each volume. Volume 32 contained reviews on the following: polyclonal B-cell activators; primed lymphocyte typing in man; protein A and related receptors; and regulation of lymphoid tumour cells. All reviews have large bibliographies; some have as many as 300 citations.

Immunological Reviews first appeared in 1961 as *Transplantation Reviews* — a fairly restrictive title in view of the general immunological nature of its contents. As many as three or four hardback volumes are published every year, each containing a number of topical reviews, all well cited. The esteem of this series is best judged by the fact that it is itself widely cited by other series, which is unusual for a secondary information source.

From the Elsevier group of publishers come two fairly similar monograph series: indeed it is very difficult to distinguish between the two in terms of subject coverage. *Developments in Immunology* is the oldest — it began in 1978 — and reached volume 17 with a 600-page review on 'Current concepts in human immunology and cancer immunomodulation' (1982). In fact most of the monographs in this series contain in excess of 400 pages. *Research Monographs in Immunology* started in 1980: volume 1 was entitled *Delayed hypersensitivity* (1980); volume 2 *Mitogenic lymphocyte transformation* (1980); volume 3 *Monoclonal antibodies and T-cell hybridomas* (1981) and volume 4 *Immunopharmacology* (1982).

It is, perhaps, surprising that Annual Review Inc. should have only very recently turned its attention to immunology in view of the immense popularity of the subject. (A compilation of articles reprinted from other Annual Reviews was published in 1980.) In 1983 the first volume of *Annual Review of Immunology* was published, containing 21 thirty-page reviews covering all main areas of the subject with large bibliographies, some having up to 200 references.

Two identically named series are published by the two major publishers in the field: Academic Press and Marcel Dekker. *Immunology*, by Dekker, reached volume 18 in 1982 with a review of 'Tumor immunity in prognosis'. *Immunology*, by Academic Press, is a series of monographs, each on various aspects of the field. 'Idiotypes and lymphocytes' was the subject of the 1981 volume.

Other serials covering the whole field of immunology include: *Comprehensive Immunology*, which reached volume 9 in 1982 with 'The immunology of human infection'; *Contemporary Topics in Molecular Immunology*; and the recently ceased *Essays in Fundamental Immunology*.

For the clinicians and those working in hospital laboratories, *Clinics in Immunology and Allergy* provides an overview of many areas of autoimmunity and immunology in general. The topics of the 1983 volumes were: Thymic Hormones; Immunological Intervention in Medicine I; and Natural Mechanism in Immunity. Each volume contains about a dozen chapters on various aspects of the individual topic. *Current Topics in Immunology* is also aimed at the medical specialist. Volume 15, published in 1981, described the immunology of skin diseases.

A number of the reviews are concerned solely with the sub-disciplines of allergy and hypersensitivity. The oldest, *Progress in Allergy,* was published for the first time in 1939 and has appeared on an irregular basis since; 'Immunity and concomitant immunity in infectious diseases' was the subject of the most recent volume published in 1982. Other series covering similar ground are: *Annual Review of Allergy, American Lectures in Allergy and Immunology* and *Monographs in Allergy.*

Immunology's practical nature is reflected in the mass of information accumulating on techniques and methods. *Methods in Immunology and Immunochemistry* has attempted to review much of this work since it was first published in 1967. 'Agglutination complement, neutralization and inhibition' (1977) and 'Antigen/antibody reactions *in vivo*' (1976) are examples of two of the older volumes. The first volume of a new series (1982), *Techniques in Immunochemistry,* contained 12 reviews on subjects including peroxidase methods, immunoelectron microscopy and tissue preparation. Immunochemical techniques are also dealt with in the series *Methods in Enzymology.* Volumes 70, 73, 74, 84, 92 and 93 comprise a mini-series within a series, entitled *Immunochemical techniques,* covering various aspects of this field including *Monoclonal antibodies and immunoassay methods* (volume 92). *Practical Methods in Clinical Immunology,* first published in 1980, included in 1983 a volume on *The immunological investigation of human virus diseases.*

Information relating to tumour immunology has traditionally been found in *Advances in Cancer Research* and *Progress in Cancer Research and Therapy.* However, since 1981 immunology has had its own series entitled *Human Cancer Immunology,* which has featured *Immune complexes and plasma exchange in cancer patients* (1981), *Suppressor cells in human cancer* (1982) and *Natural killer cells* (1982).

Two series in immunopathology, *Immunopathology* and the *Menarini Series on Immunopathology,* represent the proceedings of the International Symposia on Immunopathology and conferences organized by the Menarini Foundation respectively.

Advances in Veterinary Immunology is documented by the editors of the journal *Veterinary Immunology and Immunopathology.* It comprises an annual special issue of the journal and contains reviews in the major areas of veterinary immunology.

Developments in Biological Standardization, formerly *Progress in Immunobiological Standardization,* first published in 1955, covers the applied aspects of immunology such as vaccination and standardization.

Three specialist series are *The Antigens,* published first in 1973; *Lymphokines,* which despite its youth (it was first published in 1980) has already amassed a total of eight volumes; and *Interferon,* which began in 1979 and reached volume 5 in 1984: Gresser has edited all volumes so far.

A large number of serials carry a significant amount of immunology, but not exclusively that subject. *Current Topics in Microbiology and Immunology,* which may appear as often as six times a year, usually devotes one volume a year to an immunological topic: *Natural resistance to tumours and viruses* (1981, volume 92). Once known as *Bibliotheca Microbiologia, Contributions to Microbiology and Immunology* is a more irregularly appearing serial; volume 7 was entitled 'From parasitic infection to parasitic disease' (1982). *Advances in Experimental Medicine and Biology* appeared in two volumes in 1982; both concerning immunological subjects, they were: *Immunology of proteins and peptides* (volume 150); and *In vivo immunology — histophysiology of the lymphoid system* (volume 151).

5.3 BOOKS

Tracing and locating immunology books (*see* bibliography entries 270–291)

Book reviews

Obtaining awareness of new books in the field — there are around two hundred immunology titles published annually, from what appears to be as many outlets, and probably five times that number from immediately related disciplines — is probably the most difficult task. The information generally reaches many people through the book review or 'books received' columns of the journals they subscribe to or read regularly (scanning publishers' catalogues and browsing through specialist bookshops or the new-book shelves of specialist libraries are other very popular and pleasurable methods). Unfortunately, within the field of immunology itself few journals provide a reviewing facility. Those that do take seriously their responsibility for reviewing the literature include: *Immunology Today*, which provides the most comprehensive service by reviewing close to a hundred books a year and listing the same number again; *International Archives of Allergy* (40 a year reviewed); and *Journal of Immunological Methods* (30–40 reviewed). Probably many people in the field turn to the general scientific magazines for news and reviews of recently published books. *Science* and *Nature* both cover immunological books in similar numbers: around a dozen per year, and these of course would be the most important of those published.

While reading the book review columns of journals is a rather pleasant and painless way of keeping in touch with new books — and one which offers undoubtedly the greatest critical information — there can be no guarantee that all books will be reviewed or even listed. Because of the sheer number of books coming out, and the pressures on journal space, the coverage of the book literature by journals is inevitably selective. In such an interdisciplinary field, however, the real difficulty for the user must be in determining where a book review is likely to appear, for any number of immunology, medical, veterinary and biological journals could prove a likely outlet.

One way of minimizing the risk of missing a book review, and it is a way which does not require a great deal of effort, is to use a service that brings together the reviews published throughout a large number of journals (typically 300 or so). Probably the most widely available of such services is *Book Review Index,* which is available in both hard-copy and machine-readable (on DIALOG) forms. Although general in its coverage, it has since its inception in 1969 indexed approximately 150 reviews of immunology books. It indexes the book review columns of 380 journals and provides about 15 immunology titles per year. The books covered are either those with a potentially wide appeal, or those reviewed by popular journals like *Nature* or *Science*. Its popular bias is best illustrated by the fact that most of the reviews of books on allergies concern themselves with cooking or diet.

Less widely available, but more specialist in coverage, is *Index to Book Reviews in the Sciences* published monthly by the Institute of Scientific Information.

Abstracting and indexing services

Abstracting and indexing services, while mainly in the business of drawing attention to journal articles, do sometimes cover books, albeit selectively, and rather a long time after they have been published. Edited collections of papers or proceedings, with their 'journal-like' format and serial nature, tend to obtain best treatment. *Immunological Abstracts* provides the most comprehensive treatment of books, covering 50 or so of them a year. Accessing *Immunological Abstracts* on-line, through the *Life Sciences Collection* database on DIALOG, is to be recommended, for a facility is offered which enables a search to be conducted for books only. Indeed it is possible to search for the variant forms of the book (i.e. edited collections, conference proceedings and monographs). The immunology section alone contains 2000 references to books of all kinds, nearly 150 of them classified as monographs.

Medline used to be an invaluable source for monographs until 1981; since then their coverage has been discontinued. About 35 immunological books used to be indexed every year. These books are of course still on the database and may be retrieved.

BIOSIS Abstracts/RRM (Reports, Reviews, Meetings) provides content summaries in English for research reports and books in biology and biomedicine. This service, together with *Biological Abstracts*, is held on-line on DIALOG and is known in this form as *BIOSIS Previews*. It is not, unfortunately, possible to search the file by document form, neither can the search be confined to the RRM section. So perhaps here is a case for using it in its printed form.

Excerpta Medica covers books, but here too it is not possible to limit a database search to monographs.

Publishers' catalogues

The best sources for the most up-to-date information are publishers' catalogues and trade bibliographies. Not only do they provide the earliest notification of a book's publication, but they also provide advance notice — generally up to six months — of a book's impending publication.

Prolific publishers of immunological books include CRC Press, Dekker, Churchill Livingstone, Blackwell, Academic Press, Plenum, Elsevier and Kluwer. Some publishers' catalogues are fairly sophisticated affairs, with books arranged by special classification (Oxford University Press) or subject heading (Blackwell Scientific), and fairly lengthy summaries of their contents furnished (CRC). Some, like Wiley's, are even being offered on-line (via DIALOG), with a special alerting service electronically notifying users when titles in their sphere of interest appear. Blackwells, currently listing around 35 immunology titles, and Academic are two of the biggest publishers, with both boasting substantial catalogues (Academic's exceeding 300 pages!). Publishers' catalogues generally provide much more detail on the content of books than the conventional library listing services such as *British National Bibliography* and furthermore present the data in a far more digestible and browsable form. Publishers' catalogues are of course free and, once one is on a mailing list, will be forwarded automatically (somehow their arrival by post makes them an even more inviting source of book information). To make it easier for the individual to examine and purchase books, publishers like CRC offer their titles on an approval basis and will accept credit and payment (thus avoiding problems of currency conversion, etc.).

A fairly complete list of publishers specializing in the biological, medical and veterinary sciences can be found in Cassell's and the Publishers Association's *Directory of Publishing*. A more roundabout route to finding relevant publishers, but one yielding more specific data, is to go to the appropriate subject headings in listing tools like *Subject Guide to Books in Print* and *British National Bibliography* and identify the names of the publishers active in the field. Their addresses may be obtained — depending on which side of the Atlantic you are on — from the directory of publishers appended to *Books in Print* or *British Books in Print*. For those living outside the UK or USA, or those seeking an address for publishers outside these two countries, the *International ISBN Publishers' Directory* would serve them well.

Trade bibliographies

Because immunology books may emanate from any one of a large number of publishers, it is sometimes preferable to consult reference works that list together the entire produce of the publishing trade. Two such lists — both in fiche and hard-copy form and very popular — are *British Books in Print* and the US equivalent *Books in Print*. As books are listed alphabetically by author and title, these works are outwardly of little value to those searching for immunology books where the details are not known. However both provide keyword entries, albeit rather haphazardly. Words are taken from the title and rely entirely upon the accuracy of the book's title in portraying its contents. The fiche editions of both should be preferred as they offer a monthly appraisal of immunology books in print and new titles to come (three months' notice is commonly provided), whereas the hard copy provides such a service only on an annual basis.

The American *Books in Print* has a sister publication that is probably of more use to the immunologist: *Subject Guide to Books in Print* is an annual publication which is essentially a rearranged form of the aforesaid bibliography. Books are listed under a large number of subject headings (based upon Library of Congress practice) which are themselves arranged alphabetically. Immunology books are mainly listed under the heading 'Immunology', although some may be listed under 'Cancer' and other subjects in which immunological techniques are used (i.e. 'Enzymology'). About 730 immunology books can be located under these various headings; of these 80 were published in 1982.

Two other popular bibliographies from the same publisher as *Books in Print* are useful: *Scientific and Technical Books and Serials in Print* and *Medical Books and Serials in Print*. Both constitute a selection of documents from *Books in Print* and *Ulrich's International Periodical Directory*, and both are published annually in a handy one-volume reference form. The drawing together of serials and books on a particular topic has obvious attractions to the user. Their ease of use is considerably enhanced by the adoption of an alphabetical classified approach, which means that readers can quickly find the immunology books and serials — *Medical Books and Serials in Print* lists 55 000 books and nearly 10 000 serials.

It is probably most convenient, and certainly quicker, to use *Books in Print* and its various offshoots — *Subject Guide to Books in Print, Subject Guide to Forthcoming Books, Scientific and Technical Books in Print* and *Medical Books in Print* — in their on-line form on DIALOG. A search of this one source — called *Books in Print* too — is the equivalent to searching the latest issues of all the aforementioned publications, and furthermore one can develop a more flexible and effective search strategy based upon a combination of title words and Library of Congress headings.

As of writing it has been announced that *British Books in Print* (*BBIP*) is to go on BLAISE-Line, where it will prove a very useful supplement to *British National*

Bibliography. It will be possible for documents to be located using the sophisticated subject search keys of *BNB* and then be matched up with the latest price and publication status information from *BBIP*; it is possible already to do the equivalent operation in DIALOG where *LC Marc* offers the sophisticated subject retrieval and *BIP* the latest price and availability information. *BBIP* has no equivalent to *BIP*'s *Subject Guides*; instead for a subject approach to trade material one needs to consult *Whitaker's Classified Monthly Book List*, although the subject approach is only offered at the very general level of Medical Science and Natural Science.

Both *BIP* and *BBIP* are weak on their coverage of: unbound, free or cheap publications; government documents; textbooks; and research/academic publications (for these one needs to turn to the non-trade library-produced tools reviewed in the next section).

Non-trade bibliographic tools produced by libraries

For the coverage of immunological books there is probably no better source than the quarterly-published *Current Catalog* of the National Library of Medicine, arguably the most important medical library in the field. (More current data are obtainable through the weekly *NLM Current Catalog Proof Sheets* available from the US Medical Library Association.) Material — much of it in foreign languages — is arranged by the NLM Classification Scheme. Under this scheme Immunology books are scattered, normally to be found under QW 504, Q 1 and QR 181. Retrospective searching is facilitated by annual and quinquennial cumulations. Not widely available in its print form in Europe (though at $38.75 an annual subscription there is little financial excuse), it is however available in its on-line form, called *Catline*, on BLAISE-Link. *Catline* contains not only monographs but serials and technical reports as well, catalogued by the NLM since 1965. Retrospective conversion of the pre-1965 catalogue means that eventually the whole of the NLM *Catalog* might be available on-line. *Catline* contains 500 000 records and is updated weekly. Subject searching can be conducted through MESH headings. At less than $30 per hour access to the file is very cheap indeed.

When discussing book listing services one is inevitably led to talking about the giant on-line databases that have so recently been created through the rapid accumulation, on computer, of national bibliographies and individual library catalogues. The phenomenal success of the OCLC database, which now contains some 7 500 000 book records, and the *REMARC* programme, by which records of 5 000 000 of Library of Congress's pre-1967 published books have been put on-line (in little over three years) suggests that the day is not far off when all the world's books can be located through one gigantic database, to which everyone has access. Fortunately for the information seeker these giant files are no longer discriminating between document forms; audiovisual material, reports, books, dissertations and proceedings may all be located side by side in one single file. One hopes that users will no longer have to entangle themselves with the variant definitions of monographs employed by the various bibliographies. Finally, most of these databases do not just stop at furnishing the user with a bibliographic description of the desired works; they will, via their automatic document delivery programmes, supply the document also. This, together with the portability of modern-day on-line terminals, opens up the intriguing prospect of the immunology user never having to step into the library (unless he so wishes of course!).

For simply checking the details of a publication when the author or title is known, or for seeking North American locations for a particular book, OCLC has no peer; its sheer size guarantees that the probability of location will be high: included on the database are the holdings of over 2000 North American libraries, amongst which are the major US biomedical collections such as the National Library of Medicine. At present the value of OCLC is somewhat limited because no provision is made for a subject search. The method of searching via 'keys' derived from letters in the author's name and/or book title can initially confuse the searcher used to the natural-language-based systems like DIALOG, but is easily learnt, is less tiresome, and is often more effective for the simple bibliographic checking task. OCLC is available in Europe. *BLCMP* — another co-operative venture providing locations, but no subject approach — is a useful supplementary tool for UK users. Although not yet accessible on-line to the public, BLCMP holdings are available on monthly-produced fiche.

A subject search for US biomedical books can best be done on the Library of Congress's (LC) *Marc* databases. The *LC Marc* databases may be accessed on a number of on-line systems (DIALOG, BLAISE-Line and Orbit) but for simplicity the discussion here is limited to DIALOG, even though a more sophisticated subject approach might be obtained by using it via BLAISE. On DIALOG all Library of Congress holdings are available on just two databases: *REMARC* (1897–1967; to 1978 in the cases of some foreign-language material) and *LC Marc* (1968–); the immunology searcher will mainly be concerned with the latter, which now contains close to two million records of books from virtually all countries. The file can be searched in a large number of ways: by descriptor (LC subject heading words), any words taken from the document's title, as well as author, series, publication date, document form (i.e. catalogue) and classification number (Dewey and Library of Congress). The search may also be limited to either English or non-English records. For immunology the find is always a rich one; thus the text word immunology alone yields 868 books, the descriptor immunology retrieves 634, and even a very specific search for the presence of four terms — practical, methods, clinical and immunology — in a single document, yields over half-a-dozen references. Dissertations, proceedings, government publications, reports and research monographs, as well as the traditional book, are all to be found on the LC databases. The database, which is incidentally one of the cheapest DIALOG files to search, is updated monthly and the bibliographic description provided for each document is a very full and helpful one. The product of the search can be sorted on-line or off-line in classified, author or date order, for little extra cost. For those without on-line facilities *MARCFICHE* provides much the same detail but not of course the array of access points or the sorting facilities. However it is possible to search on LC number, and in this form LC cataloguing is very portable and cheap.

Other very valuable bibliographic sources published in the USA, but not confined solely to its output, are the *National Union Catalog* (*NUC*) and *RLIN*, the Research Libraries Group's on-line Bibliographic Data Base.

The *NUC*, covering the holdings of 1500 North American libraries in addition to the LC, is even broader in compass than the *LC Marc* database. It is now only available in fiche form, which does make it much more accessible and useful to European libraries. In this form too, subject access is provided for the first time — the subject entries are created from LC subject headings. Issued monthly, the revamped *NUC* consists of one master register in accession number with cumulating name, title, series and subject indexes. At an annual subscription of $350 the *NUC* catalogue must represent excellent value for money. In fiche form the *Catalog* is only searchable back to 1983.

The Research Libraries Information Network (RLIN) provides for, among many other things, on-line bibliographic retrieval. The particular relevance of the *Network* for immunologists lies in: (a) the quality and strength of the research collections contributing their records to the database — Johns Hopkins, the University of California at Berkeley, Stanford University, Rutgers and Yale (251 000 records from the National Library of Medicine and the United States Government Printing Office are being added in 1983/84; and *LC Marc* data are fed continuously into the database); and (b) the range of subject search keys by which the data may be accessed (i.e. by Library of Congress, Dewey and National Library of Medicine class numbers; subject phrase; and title word phrase). The bibliographic database is itself divided into six sub-files, one of which is the book file containing seven million records. The database is continuously updated, costs around $60 an hour to search, and can be accessed either using direct-dial telephoning or the services of TYMNET.

For seekers of UK immunological monographs the situation is somewhat simpler, for there is really only one comprehensive and effective search medium — the *British National Bibliography*, known as *UK MARC* in its machine-readable form. For all but browsing, where the hard-copy form with its classified format (albeit Dewey, which scatters immunological publications around the major disciplines) and more importantly, excellent subject index, with its effective network of 'see' and 'see also' references, the machine variant (on BLAISE) is always to be preferred. The sheer size of the database (back to 1950), and lack of cumulation (a search covering the last two years' output of monographs for instance) might involve consulting a dozen separate issues/volumes) makes manual searching tiresome, lengthy and very ineffective. Even in machine-readable form we do not, unfortunately, have one look-up point, the data being held on three files: 1950–70, 1971–76, 1977–; although to the immunological searcher, essentially interested in a very up-to-the-minute literature, the search will in effect only involve on file — the latest one. In theory, because of copyright law, all books published in the UK should be present on the database (in practice grey literature like reports and proceedings still proves elusive) and generally a wide range of monographs are indeed listed. However the major strength of *BNB*, and *UK MARC* in particular, lies in its excellent subject retrieval capabilities — items may be located via Dewey 19th class numbers (616.07918/9, 636.089 and 574.2918/9 proving among the most useful), UDC class mark (612.017), Library of Congress classification numbers (QR 181 is the most productive), Library of Congress subject heading, subject word, précis word, and SIN number. The latter is a particularly powerful and time-saving retrieval device if you happen to alight upon a précis descriptor string that exactly matches your needs. Thus the number for Bowry's *Immunology simplified* is 0016454, and a search based on this number retrieves 41 documents including such relevant and related titles as Schwartz's *Compendium of immunology* and Clark's *The experimental foundations of modern immunology*. It is of course also possible to search by any word in the title. Document-form retrieval is also particularly effective, with the ability to call up dictionaries, encyclopedias, statistics and yearbooks, for instance.

Immunology books

What makes a good scientific book? According to *Nature* (1982), good books possess the following two characteristics. First, they are written by a single author who is commonly a practising lecturer and able to transfer the enthusiasm he generates in the lecture room to the page. Secondly, the book has a 'grand sweep' — the selection and emphasis of the material is not what would be recommended by an academic committee 'brooding' about the exact balance of some student course.

Proof of these ideas exists in immunology, where the truly outstanding books do possess the above characteristics. Foremost of these is Ivan Roitt's *Essential immunology* (1984), which first appeared in 1971 and is now in its fifth edition — that in itself a testament to its undoubted popularity. It is no overstatement to say that this textbook has influenced the nature of what is taught, rather than slavishly following established practices. Much the same could be said for *Immunology at a glance* by Playfair (1982). This book is not only unique in format — consisting of a series of large, explicit diagrams (hence the name) — but is also one of the rare immunology texts that could be read by the interested layman as well as undergraduates in the biomedical sciences.

Two other books which deserve special mention are *General immunology* by Cooper (1982) and *Immunology: the science of self–non self discrimination* by Klein (1982). Both are 'mould-breakers', and Klein's has the added distinction of being controversial — reviewers either loved or hated it.

All the aforementioned books are introductory in character, aimed largely at students and those in related disciplines who require a basic grounding in immunology. As the subject becomes more complex however, the multi-author, sometimes multi-volume, tome becomes the norm. Style takes a back seat in these publications, which may more accurately be termed treatises. These treatises allow for an extended and comprehensive coverage of the subject by a group of experts (sometimes as many as fifty!) representing the specialized disciplines. In immunology these works form the bulk of the monograph literature.

In this section the following types of publications will be considered together because they fundamentally share the same purpose: monographs, manuals, treatises and one-off proceedings. Selection is never easy in science because of the general uniformity of quality and content of its publications. The problem is compounded in immunology by the sheer number of books in print — at least 500; and this total is being added to at a rate of 80 a year. The books included in the following section are essentially mainstream texts which have been published in the last five years, with few exceptions. For convenience they are divided into broad categories although inevitably in such a diverse field there is some overlapping. Additional titles are listed in the bibliography.

General (*see* bibliography entries 292–313)

The most popular text for undergraduates of all immunological persuasions, be they microbiology, medical or veterinary students, is Roitt's *Essential immunology* (1984). The current (fifth) edition is considerably revised and covers the entire field, in 400 pages. There are new sections on monoclonal antibodies, idiotypic networks, laser nephrometry and fluorescent activated cell sorter systems. *Immunology at a glance* by Playfair (1982) is the perfect antidote to much of the immunology literature: its unusual format enables the reader to grasp the basic principles by studying a series of large, explicit diagrams each dealing with a particular topic. Topics covered include natural immunity, adaptive immunity, undesirable effects of immunity, and altered immunity. Another diagrammatic presentation of immunology is found in a more recent book called *The chain of immunology*, by Feinberg and Jackson (1983). It is twice the size of Playfair's book but even then has only 86 pages. It depicts the events leading to the immune response, in a series of sequential charts. Klein's controversial book *Immunology: the science of self–non self discrimination* (1982) attempts to cover the entire field of immunology. The work is divided into four parts. The first part covers the history of the subject; the second part describes the structure of the organs, receptors and molecules involved in immunology; the third part, the mechanisms of the macrophages and B- and T-lymphocytes; and the fourth part concerns the synthesis. *General immunology* by Cooper (1982) is aimed at the biology undergraduate rather than the medical student. It is well written and has good illustrations.

Basic and clinical immunology (4th edn, 1982), edited by Stites *et al.*, was first published in 1976 and since then has been translated into seven other languages. It is divided into basic immunology, immunological laboratory tests and clinical immunology. In addition it has a useful glossary of terms, acronyms and abbreviations used in immunology. The editors intend to update with biennial editions. *Immunology*, edited by Bach (2nd edn, 1982) has been translated and updated from the original French text published a few years ago. Although it is over a thousand pages long, the £52 price tag will place it out of the range of most students and many libraries. Developed from lectures given at Harvard Medical School, *Textbook of immunology*, by Benacernaf and Unanue (1979), is an introduction-cum-review of immunology for students, teachers and workers.

The immune system, edited by Steinberg and Lefkovits (1981), is a tribute to the work of Niels Jerne. Its two volumes entitled *Past and future* and *The present* cover advances in basic immunology made possible through the work of this eminent immunologist. *Immunology — benchmarks papers in microbiology*, edited by Golub (1981), in two volumes, is another historical account of the development of immunology. Part 1 deals with 'cell interaction' and part 2 with 'regulation'.

Other good texts covering basic immunology are: *Fundamentals of immunology* by Bier *et al.* (1981); *Principles of immunology* (2nd edn, 1979) edited by Rose *et al.*; *The immune system — a course on the molecular and cellular basis of immunity* by McConnell *et al.* (2nd edn, 1981); *Textbook of immunology: an introduction to immunochemistry and immunobiology* by Barret (4th edn, 1983); *Fundamental immunology*, edited by Paul (1983) and *Experimental foundations of modern immunology* by Clark (1980).

History of immunology (see bibliography entries 314–317)

Many immunology texts precede their account of basic and clinical immunology with an introductory chapter on the history and development of the subject. Some good examples are: *Immunology for students of medicine*, by Humphrey and White (3rd edn, 1970); *The science of self*, by Wilson (1972); *Immunology: the science of self–non-self discrimination*, by Klein (1982) and *General immunology* by Cooper (1982).

Volume 1 of *The immune system* (subtitled: *Past and future*), edited by Steinberg and Lefkovits (1981), surveys the evolution of fundamental concepts in immunology, and is largely a tribute to one immunologist: Niels Jerne.

Immunology: benchmark papers in microbiology, edited by Golub (1981), is a collection of annotated papers that have made a significant contribution to the development of immunology.

For the more erudite, the best and most recent account is to be found in the journal *Cellular Immunology* (1982–83). It is written in four parts by Arthur Silverstein of the Johns Hopkins University and entitled: 'History of immunology: development of the concept of immunologic specificity'. As well as covering the theoretical and practical developments, it provides a valuable insight into the characters of early immunologists.

Allergy, autoimmunity and hypersensitivity (*see* bibliography entries 318–328)

Current perspectives in allergy represents volume 1 of *Contemporary Issues in Clinical Immunology and Allergy* edited by Goetzl and Kay (1982). It provides general practitioners with an update and perspective of clinical and research data in allergic disease; how many other volumes are to come is uncertain at this time. *Immunological and clinical aspects of allergy* is aimed at a similar audience. This book, edited by Lessof (1981), reflects the large increase in our basic knowledge of the allergic mechanisms and aims to bridge the gap between basic science and its clinical application. A more specialist text, *Nasal allergy*, by Mygind (1979), considers the immunology of the nose.

Autoimmunity, by Talal (1977), while perhaps a little old now, is still the standard text in the field. It is divided into genetic, immunological, viral and clinical aspects. Two books devote themselves solely to the immunology of the endocrine system. They are *Autoimmunity in the endocrine system*, by Volpé (1981), and *Autoimmune aspects of endocrine disorders*, edited by Pinchera *et al.* (1981). *Modulation of autoimmunity and disease: the penicillamine experience*, edited by Maini and Berry (1981), contains 41 reports and seven edited discussions from a workshop on D-penicillamine — a drug used for arthritis and other inflammatory conditions.

Pseudo-allergic reactions. Involvement of drugs and chemicals, edited by Dukor *et al.* (1980), presents 11 reports on the pseudo-allergic reactions, covering genetic aspects and anaphylactic reactions.

The allergy encyclopaedia, edited by the Asthma and Allergy Foundation of America (1981) is, unusually, written for the patient (really the American patient) by nine distinguished doctors.

Due for publication in 1984, *Allergy: principles and practice*, edited by Middleton and others in two volumes, focuses on the developments in allergy over the last 10 years, and on the variety of clinical states dealt with by the allergist.

Cellular immunology and cytotoxicity (*see* bibliography entries 329–347)

For those interested in the historical perspective of this field *Cellular immunology (selected readings and critical commentary)*, edited by Sato and Gefter (1981), is recommended. It consists of a collection of classical papers covering the major areas of cellular immunology. Each section is preceded by an introductory chapter.

Two complementary and highly recommended publications are both compiled from recently commissioned articles appearing in the journal *Immunology Today*. *B-lymphocytes today*, edited by Inglis (1982), contains 27 reviews covering immunoglobulin genes and antibody synthesis, activation of B-cells, their markers, and their function in disease. *T-lymphocytes today*, edited by Inglis (1983), describes: genes and receptors; ontogeny and education; activation and regulation; effector mechanisms; and disorder of function. Both these reasonably priced books can be read by students, teachers and research workers.

Clinical cellular immunology: molecular and therapeutic reviews, edited by Luderer and Weetal (1982), provides a structured review of both clinical and non-clinical cell-mediated immunity.

Phagocytes and cellular immunity, edited by Gadebusch (1979), deals with the destructive role of mononuclear and polymorphonuclear leukocytes and the constructive properties of macrophages influencing cellular immunity and humoral antibody response.

Bringing together both types of lymphocytes in one volume is *T- and B-lymphocytes: recognition and function*, edited by Bach *et al.* (1979). This book represents the proceedings of an ICN–UCLA Symposium on Molecular Biology.

NK cells and other natural effector cells, edited by Herberman (1982), covers immune effector systems ranging from studies of their nature, regulation and mechanisms of action, to their role in host resistance, their modulation by therapeutic intervention, and alteration of their activity in disease.

Clinical immunology (*see* bibliography entries 348–357)

The standard reference text for medical students is *Clinical aspects of immunology*, edited by Lachmann and Peters (1982), now in its fourth, fully revised edition. The £90 price for the two-volume set, however, means most students will borrow it from libraries rather than buy their own copies. The 70 or so contributors of 'Gell and Coombs' as it has become known (after the original editors) combine to produce 11 sections covering: physiological systems of the allergic response; advances in immunological technology; allergic mechanisms of tissue damage; organ based immunology; tumour immunology; and immunology of infection. Of similar size and doing a similar job is *Immunology in medicine: a comprehensive guide to clinical immunology*, by Holborow and Reeves (1983), now in its second edition. Eight introductory chapters on the basics of the immune system are followed by a more detailed examination of the role of the immune system in disease, system disorders, and the lymphoproliferative and malignant diseases.

Immunology in clinical medicine, by Turk and Collins (3rd edn, 1978), is directed at medical students, and costs just over £5 for 265 pages. The first four chapters are concerned with basic immunology, while the rest of the book is devoted to actual disease processes. To supplement the medical teaching, the student may also buy *Lecture notes on clinical immunology* by Reeves (1981). *Clinical immunology* (2nd edn), by Richter (1982), contains detailed discussion of the interpretation and significance of immunological tests. It is intended for physicians or clinical research workers.

The self-explanatory *Clinical immunology update: review for physicians*, edited by Franklin (1983), covers: subsets of T-cells in man; analyses of leukaemic states; immune complexes and autoimmune diseases involving the kidneys and connective tissues; and allergy and its effect. The editor intends to issue biennial editions. *Immunization in clinical practice*, edited by Fulginiti (1982), is subtitled 'A useful guideline to vaccines, sera and immune globulins in clinical practice'.

The *Handbook of immunology for students and house staff*, edited by Fikrig (1982), is an easily accessible source of information on clinical immunology and emphasizes treatment throughout.

Developmental immunology (see bibliography entries 358–360)

A great deal of interest has focused on this new area, and this has been reflected in the recent publication of three similar books: *The CRC handbook of immunology in aging*, edited by Kay and Makinodan (1981); *Developmental immunology: clinical problems and aging*, by Cooper and Brazier (1982); and *Immunology and aging*, by Fabris (1982). All concern themselves with ageing theories and development, and ageing of the immune system. In addition Kay and Makinodan's contribution includes reviews of methods for assessing the immune response during the ageing process.

Immune response and immunoglobulins (see bibliography entries 361–364)

Works on the regulation of the immune system seem to be the domain of one editor: Eli Sercarz. His three books — *Strategies of immune regulation* (1980); *The immune system: genes, receptors, signals* (1974); and *The immune system: genetics and regulation* (1978) — probably say all there is to be said on the subject. *Regulation of immune response dynamics*, edited by Delisi and Hiernaux (1982), focuses, in two volumes, on auto-anti-idiotypic regulation and T-cell regulation.

Immunoglobulin idiotypes, edited by Janeway and others (1981) — one of whom is Sercarz — represents the proceedings of a symposium held in 1981 which covered immunoglobulin genes and their products, T-cell receptors, regulation of immune response and shifting paradigms in immunology.

Immunity to infection (see bibliography entries 365–374)

A number of good, but dated, titles deal with viral immunology: *Viral immunology and immunopathology*, edited by Notkins (1975); and *Viruses and immunity*, edited by Koprowski and Koprowski (1975), provide fairly complex introductions to the field. A more recent publication is *Immunological investigation of human virus diseases*, by McLean (1983). It provides practical details of immunological techniques and a critical evaluation of their reliability and interpretation.

Parasitic diseases: volume 1, *The immunology*, edited by Mansfield (1981), is rather an expensive review of the clinical and experimental immunology of some of the major parasites: malaria, trypanosoma cruzi, schistosoma, and filarial nematodes. *Immunoparasitology: principles and methods in malaria and schistosomiasis research*, edited by Strickland and Hunter (1982), focuses on just two parasitic diseases.

Immunological aspects of infection in the fetus and newborn, edited by Lambert and Wood (1981), discusses the role of the placenta in protection from infection; development and maturation of immunity transmitted in breast milk, and the future prospects for protection.

Viral pathogenesis and immunology, by Mims and White (1984), is a very recent addition to the field. For the bacteriologist, *Bacterial infection and immunity* is written by Woolcock (1979).

Immunogenetics, human leukocyte antigen (HLA) and the major histocompatibility complex (MHC) (see bibliography entries 375–380)

Essential immunogenetics, by Williamson and Turner (1981), is a concise account of the basic facts and ideas relating to the genetics of the immune system, for students and research workers. *Frontiers in immunogenetics*, edited by Hildemann

(1981), is organized into four sections: allogenic polymorphism and immunophylogeny; genetics of immune responsiveness; immunodifferentiation and development; and immunogenetics and disease. A more detailed treatise by Hildemann (1981) is contained in *Comprehensive immunogenetics*.

HLA and disease, by Braun (1979), reviews the human leukocyte antigen system of man, the historical development techniques employed, genetics, and clinical applicability. *HLA without tears*, by Miller and Rodey (1981), is a more introductory account. *The role of the major histocompatibility complex in immunobiology*, edited by Dorf (1982), takes a wider perspective of this complex area.

Immunogenetics, by Zaleski et al. (1983), describes the basic principles of genetics before discussing in more detail immunoglobulins, blood groups, MHC and cell surface allo-antigens of nucleated cells. It is modestly priced.

Immunohaematology (*see* bibliography entries 381–382)

An introduction to immunohaematology, by Bryant (2nd edn, 1982), includes new material on quality control, HLA and blood groups, as well as expanded coverage of blood typing, complement and antibody identification. *Immunotherapy: a guide to immunoglobulin prophylaxis and therapy*, edited by Nyedegger (1982), provides basic medical knowledge of immunoglobulins and their use in intravenous infusions.

Immunopathology (*see* bibliography entries 383–401)

Advances in immunopathology, edited by Weigle (1981), covers molecular and cellular events in the immune response; mediators of inflammation; and immunovirology and immunopathology. A cheaper and smaller alternative to the above is *The biology of immunologic disease*, edited by Dixon and Fisher (1983). The 39 contributors cover five main topics: the development of immunological potential; primary pathology of lymphoid tissues; mediators of immunological theory; immunological diseases; and therapeutic approaches to immunological diseases. In the same area, Dixon and Fisher are preparing a new text entitled *Immunopathology* (1984).

Immunological investigation of connective tissue disease, by Glynn and Reading (1981), is a small book illustrating how far laboratory tests have progressed in this field since the recognition of rheumatoid factor and the lupus erythematosus cell. *Immune mechanisms in renal disease*, edited by Cummings and Michael (1983), is a collection of papers covering 'the cutting edge' of research in kidney immunopathology.

Immunological aspects of liver disease, edited by Thomas et al. (1982), focuses on hepatic immunopathology; *Immunology of diabetes*, edited by Irvine (1981), considers this pancreatic defect; *Immunology of the human placenta*, edited by Klopper (1982), examines this complex organ; and *Immunology of inflammation*, edited by Ward (1983), describes the primary immune response.

Finally, *Immunologic considerations in toxicology*, edited by Sharma and Street (1980), is an account of the rapidly emerging field of immunotoxicology.

Interferon (*see* bibliography entries 402–405)

Interferon: a primer, by Friedman (1981), eases the reader into this topical subject by describing the basic properties of these proteins. For those wishing to know a little more, there are five volumes on the subject by Gresser. They are: *Interferon 1 1979* (1979); *Interferon 2 1980* (1981); *Interferon 3 1981* (1982); *Interferon 1982: Volume*

4 (1982); and *Interferon 1984: Volume 5* (1984). *Interferon and cancer,* edited by Sikora (1983), examines the effects of interferon on the growth of tumours.

The proceedings of a UCLA symposium on molecular and cellular biology is contained in a volume entitled *Interferons,* edited by Merigan and Friedman (1982). It covers: recombinant DNA production of interferon; the biology of interferon; factors relevant to the clinical application of interferon; and clinical studies with interferon.

Monoclonal antibodies (hybridoma technology)   (*see* bibliography entries 406–417)

For those without any practical knowledge of monoclonal antibodies, *Monoclonal antibodies: production and maintenance,* by Løvborg (1982), provides a good starting point. It is a manual and guide to hybridoma theory and practical techniques, with useful appendices, a glossary of terms and a limited bibliography — packed into just 66 pages. Another introductory text, *Monoclonal antibodies,* by Sikora and Smedley (1984), explains what monoclonal antibodies are and how to produce them, and discusses their application.

Monoclonal antibodies in clinical medicine, edited by McMichael and Fabre (1982), is a more erudite offering. It begins with historical aspects and general principles, and is then arranged into 24 chapters covering all the main areas of clinical research. The use of monoclonal antibodies in diagnosis, prognosis and therapy is discussed throughout. *Monoclonal antibodies. Hybridomas: a new dimension in biological analyses,* edited by Kennett and others (1980), is a more concise account of the broad applications of monoclonal antibodies, and discusses potential uses.

Monoclonal antibodies and developments in immunoassay, edited by Albertini and Ekins (1981), discusses the significance of monoclonal antibodies in immunoassay and their use with calciotropic hormones.

Monoclonal antibodies and T-cell products, edited by Katz (1982), examines the role of both B- and T-cell hybridomas as research and diagnostic probes. Other topics include application to autoimmunity and molecular diversity of retroviruses, but at £65 for 176 pages it is very poor value.

Of more specialist interest for neurologists is *Monoclonal antibodies to neural antigens,* edited by McKay *et al.* (1981).

Neuroimmunology and immunopharmacology   (*see* bibliography entries 418–425)

Neuroimmunology, edited by Brockes (1982), and *Clinical neuroimmunology,* by Rose (1979), are the two main texts in this important new sub-discipline. They are both lucid and scholarly introductions to the use of immunological techniques in the study of the nervous system.

Psychoneuroimmunology, edited by Ader (1981) discusses the effect of psychosocial factors and stress on the disease and immune processes.

Immunology of nervous system infections, edited by Behan *et al.* (1983), brings together a variety of specialists from neurology, immunology, virology, and the veterinary sciences, to discuss the relationship between infection and immunology in the nervous system.

Textbook of immunopharmacology, edited by Dale and Foreman (1983), covers the mechanisms involved in the formation, release and action of the chemical mediators of inflammation and other immune reactions; it includes a chapter on drugs which modify the inflammatory immune response. Two other texts in this area are *Immunopharmacology*, edited by Rola-Pleszczynski and Sirois (1982), and *Immunopharmacology and the regulation of leukocyte function* by Webb (1982).

Techniques (including immunochemistry) (*see* bibliography entries 426–445)

The most readable account, of the dozens of books concerned with immunological techniques, is *Practical immunology* (2nd edn), by Hudson and Hay (1980). Reasonably priced and easy to follow, this revised edition includes chapters on immunoassays, hybridoma cells and monoclonal antibodies, immune complexes and parasites, isolation of immunoglobulins, and affinity chromatography. Appendices on buffers, equipment and manufacturing suppliers complete this popular book, aimed at workers in research laboratories. Similarly *Handbook of experimental immunology* (3rd edn), edited by Weir (1978) in three volumes, is a research tool, albeit an expensive one. Volume 1 covers immunochemistry, volume 2 cellular immunology, and volume 3 application of immunological methods.

Manual of clinical immunology*, edited by Rose and Friedman (2nd edn, 1980), is designed for the clinical laboratory. It contains general methods and procedures for measuring humoral and cellular factors; laboratory examination of patients with allergic and immuno-deficient diseases; immunological tests in tumour immunology; and immunoassays. At about £16 for over 1000 pages it represents value for money. Thompson's *Techniques in clinical immunology* (1981) is a concise account of the same subject, albeit with a more pronounced British emphasis.

Four books devote themselves to immunochemistry. They are: *Antibody as a tool. The applications of immunochemistry*, edited by Marchalonis and Warr (1982); *Immunochemistry in practice*, by Johnstone and Thorpe (1982); *Immunocytochemistry: practical applications in pathology and biology*, edited by Polak and Van Noorden (1983); and *Immunohistochemistry*, edited by Cuello (1983).

Transplantation, immunosuppression and immunotolerance (*see* bibliography entries 446–453)

Liver transplantation*, edited by Calne (1983), covers the study of the ability of both the organ and recipient to withstand the operation; methods of preservation, patterns of rejection, and immunosuppression. *Renal transplantation: theory and practice*, edited by Hamburger *et al.* (1981), deals with all aspects of kidney transplants. *Biology of bone marrow transplantation*, edited by Gale *et al.* (1980), represents the proceedings of a symposium on cell and molecular biology.

Cellular and molecular mechanisms of immunologic tolerance*, edited by Hraba and Hazek (1981), is divided into five sections: active mechanisms of immuno-tolerance; mechanism of immune reaction inhibition at the cellular level; cellular interaction in immuno-tolerance; transplantation tolerance; and the biological role of immuno-tolerance.

Transplantation immunology*, edited by Calne (1984), contains many new transplantation procedures, and considers both clinical work and *in vitro* experimental results.

Tumour immunology (*see* bibliography entries 454–463)

All books listed here are for the specialist — they are complex works.

Mechanisms of immunity to virus-induced cancers*, edited by Blasecki (1981), is directed primarily towards the mechanism of immunity operating in tumour rejection.

There is also a good deal of information on the immune response as measured *in vitro*. *Radiotherapy and cancer immunology*, edited by Prasad (1981), is a compilation of information on the impact of radiotherapy on the immune system of patients with various forms of cancer.

Mediation of cellular immunity in cancer by immune modifiers, edited by Chirigos *et al.* (1981), comprises a series of contributions given at a workshop on the effects of the biological response modifiers on cell-mediated immunity. *Natural cell mediated immunity against tumors*, edited by Herberman (1980), is a large and expensive work on the natural killer (NK) and related cells, charting their mechanism of cytotoxicity, immunogenetic regulation, *in vivo* and *in vitro* role and activity.

B- and T-cell tumors: biological and clinical aspects, edited by Vitetta (1983), describes the origin and classification of tumours; characteristics and regulation of T- and B-cell clones; and tumour therapy. *Immunotherapy of human cancer*, edited by Terry and Rosenberg (1982), provides a compendium of recent material on important clinical trials of immunotherapeutics in the treatment of established cancers.

Veterinary immunology (*see* bibliography entries 467–470)

Veterinary immunology, once a fairly neglected area, has recently attracted much interest. *An introduction to veterinary immunology* (2nd edn), by Tizard (1982), has been greatly revised since 1977. Major changes are found in the genetics of immunoglobulin synthesis, cellular interaction, and regulation of the immune response through the MHC. Examples of the immune system of domestic animals are cited throughout. *Advances in veterinary immunology*, by Kristensen and Antczak (1982), discusses: immunity to intracellular bacteria, immunological activities of milk, and lymphocyte markers in the pig; idiotypes and autoimmune thyroiditis in dogs; and the lymphocyte stimulation test in veterinary immunology.

Animal models of immunological processes, edited by Hay (1982), stresses the importance of *in vivo* rather than *in vitro* studies. Topics include: canine immune responses; migration patterns of lymphocytes in sheep; and mucosa-associated systems in rabbits. *Immunology and immunization of fish*, edited by Muiswinkel and Cooper (1981), is a supplement to the journal *Developmental and Comparative Immunology*, and carries the proceedings of a meeting held on immunological aspects of fish biology.

5.4 DISSERTATIONS

Introduction

Dissertations or theses do play an important, if specialist, role in the immunology information system. Their value lies mainly in the level of detail provided, particularly with regard to the methods adopted. Whereas the practical problems and real 'nitty gritty' associated with conducting experiments (at its most basic level, the washing of laboratory instruments) are not generally mentioned in research papers, they *are* included in dissertations. Therefore in many ways dissertations can be used as manuals of practice. They are valued too for the supposed originality of the material, but this is a much more contentious issue. They are also likely to be more up-to-date than journal articles.

Their detractors would argue, however, that their sheer bulk, variability in quality and ponderous style make them the last resort as an information source.

Certainly the fact that few have indexes makes it difficult to retrieve information from them quickly. None the less, the great advances that have been made in making dissertations more accessible will inevitably mean that they will become an increasingly important information source for immunologists.

Tracing and location dissertations (*see* bibliography entries 478–486)

Dissertation Abstracts International, published by University Microfilms, is probably the most widely known and available of the reference tools that provide details of recently accepted dissertations — in this case doctoral dissertations. It comes in three volumes; volume B, *The Sciences and Engineering,* and volume C, *European Abstracts,* are of interest. Very detailed abstracts (500 words) are furnished for each dissertation. Dissertations in volume B, published monthly, are mainly North American, but South American, Belgian and Finnish dissertations are also featured and are arranged under broad subject divisions for browsing. Most, but not all, immunology theses can be located under the Health Sciences subheading 'Immunology'. Within this subheading they are arranged alphabetically by author. However, the subject index (there is also an author index) must also be consulted, for about half the immunological theses can be located under the various biological sciences subject headings. The index is based upon words in the title, so care must be taken when using it. The importance of dissertations as information sources (and the productivity of US universities) is underlined by the fact that *Dissertation Abstracts* currently lists around 200 immunology dissertations per year. Most of these dissertations are abstracted about six to nine months after submission, and most can be obtained in photocopy or microfiche form from the publishers, University Microfilms. Abstracts are so long and informative (200 words is quite common) that they might sometimes serve instead of the dissertation.

Dissertation Abstracts can be accessed on-line via DIALOG, as can *American Doctoral Dissertations* (a computer-generated index, by keywords and author, to US dissertations accepted between 1861 and 1972), *Comprehensive Dissertation Index* (an annual consolidation of US and Canadian dissertations listed in *Dissertation Abstracts International*) and *Masters Abstracts* (as the title suggests, a list of master's theses, primarily American). The resultant database — *Dissertation Abstracts On-line* — provides a subject, title and author guide to virtually every dissertation accepted by an American university or college since 1861, when academic doctoral degrees were first awarded. Altogether the comprehensive dissertation index contains details of nearly 1 000 000 dissertations, of which about 2100 are of direct immunological interest. Abstracts are included for a large majority of the degrees granted after January 1980. This full-text feature enables a more thorough keyword search, scanning not only citations, but the body of each abstract as well. A subject heading approach is also possible using the descriptor code number 0982 for immunology.

For the UK, coverage of dissertations is the responsibility of two publications: *Index to Theses,* published by Aslib, and the British Library's *British Reports, Translations and Theses.* The Aslib index is a long-running one, having been published since 1950, and covers theses issued by colleges and polytechnics as well as universities. Not all universities or colleges are represented, and the only way to learn about the ·theses produced by such institutions is to go to the individual universities' lists themselves. *Index to Theses* is published twice yearly, so cannot hope to be as current as its US counterpart. In fact theses are listed as long as 18 months after submission. They are arranged by broad subject heading, immunology theses being listed under the heading Pathology and Clinical Medicine: immunology. The subject index is needed to retrieve all immunology theses, for some may be located under other headings, particularly medicine. About 15 immunology theses are listed a year, far less than the *Dissertation Abstracts* figure of 200. No summary of the content of the theses is provided in the *Index to Theses*, simply sufficient data to enable them to be traced. However, abstracts of most of these theses can be obtained from its sister publication *Abstracts of Theses*, which is available only in microfiche. Photocopies of theses can also be obtained.

British Reports, Translations and Theses is an invaluable tool as it is essentially a list of the British Library Lending Division's British thesis holdings (this library receives all the theses listed in *Dissertation Abstracts*), therefore everything that is listed can be loaned or photocopied — and obtained within a few days. Published monthly, it is much more up-to-date than the Aslib list, with theses just 6–12 months late in being announced. As its name suggests it is not just a list of theses, so one has to browse through reports and translations as well, which may of course be useful as other relevant items may also be picked up. Material is arranged by broad subject; immunology is placed under 'Clinical medicine', which is itself a subheading of 'Biological and medical sciences'. Immunology theses may also be located elsewhere in the arrangement, so the keyword index must always be consulted. Approximately 5 immunology theses are listed per issue. As the British Library has a collection of over 20 000 theses it is well worth searching retrospectively (via the annual indexes) through *British Reports, Translations and Theses*. It is possible to go back as far as 1971.

Some abstracting and indexing journals (e.g. *Immunological Abstracts*) also cover theses, but usually selectively. There are just 29 on the *Life Sciences Collection* from all biological fields.

5.5 PATENTS

Introduction (*see* bibliography entries 487–489)

In 1975 Cesar Milstein contacted the British government to ask whether a technique he and his collaborator Georges Kohler had developed should be patented because of its great commercial potential. There was no response. Consequently the two Cambridge workers went ahead and published their results in *Nature*. This action immediately barred them from receiving royalties from commercial exploitation of their discovery, hybridoma technology.

Whether or not Milstein's original work could have been patented is still hotly disputed. Some claim that as the application of standard cell fusion techniques is in wide use around the world there is nothing inherently patentable about Milstein's use of the hybridoma. Others feel that as a sufficiently novel application of the techniques, a patent might indeed have been granted. So it seemed, from a British point of view anyway, that as in the case of penicillin nearly 50 years earlier, an opportunity had been lost.

With industrial investment at $25 million in 1980, and expected to grow to $500 million in 1987 in the hybridoma research field, patenting is, indeed, a crucial issue.

The Americans have certainly not been slow in this area. Two significant patents have been granted protection by the USA and several European countries: a broad patent for monoclonals against tumour cells, granted in October 1979, and another to viral antigens in April 1980, both to Hilary Koprowski and Carlo Croce of the Wistar Institute. However the British Patent Office have ruled that the work was an obvious application of the basic hybridoma procedures, an objection which has been upheld by the British Patent Court in 1983. Similar problems have been encountered in Japan, where 27 separate challenges have been filed. Unlike the USA, which allows an inventor to apply for a patent up to a year after disclosure, Japan (like Britain and Western Europe) demands 'absolute novelty'. Those challenging the patent are basing their case largely on an article that appeared in *Nature* the day before the US patent application was filed. If the challenges are upheld Wistar would lose the Japanese market, which is the second largest pharmaceutical market in the world.

In 1980 the IUIS presented its members with a resolution critical of attempts to patent the products of hybridomas. It was proposed that hybridomas and their products should be freely accessible to all, and without restriction or patent rights.

But such moves are unlikely to stem the tide. US research centres such as Stanford, Washington, Harvard and Wisconsin universities scrutinize all products and processes emerging from research for market potential and value of patent protection; terms are then arranged with commercial companies to sell them under licence. Stanford's annual royalties on around 180 patent items exceed $600 000.

Critics of patenting fear increased secrecy interfering in scientific exchange, erosion of academic freedom, and hindrance between groups from different institutions who may be looking at related aspects of common problems.

But just what is patenting and are the above fears justified? Crespi, in his book *Patenting in the biological sciences* (1982), defines the basis of a patent as a bargain made between the inventor and the government, usually the Patent or Industrial Property Office, whereby the latter grants for a specified period a right to exclude others from exploiting the invention without the inventor's permission. For his part the inventor must make a full disclosure of the invention in a written specification which is published in due course and made available for public use freely after the specified period has terminated.

The justification for the patent system according to Crespi is threefold:

1. It encourages disclosure as against secrecy,
2. It encourages investment in research,
3. It encourages investment in production and marketing of new products.

That these points conflict so markedly with the fears of the critics of patenting indicates the complexities and misconceptions that abound in the area of patent legislation. Consequently there is a need for clear and concise guides to the world's patent systems, which clearly were not designed to cope with the developments seen in the biosciences.

Crespi's *Patenting in the biological sciences* (1982) is a practical guide for research scientists in biotechnology and the pharmaceutical and agrochemical industries. It covers the categories, the mechanism, the condition, the strategies, and enforcement of patenting; special considerations of chemical, microbiological and genetic engineering; and includes extracts from European and American patent conventions.

While there are many examples of patents given in the book, unfortunately only a few deal specifically with immunological inventions (e.g. Marek's disease vaccine).

Information sources in biotechnology, by Crafts-Lighty (1983), includes a very readable introductory account of patents and patenting, supplemented with an extensive bibliography.

On a more general level, *Patent licensing: a guide to the literature* by the British Library's Science Reference Library (December 1982) is an eight-page pamphlet arranged in four parts. The first part contains an annotated listing of a dozen books on licensing in Europe, Japan, the USA and the USSR, all fairly up-to-date, mostly post-1978. The second part is an annotated listing of nine periodicals providing information about licensing opportunities internationally. The third part gives information on official patent publications, notably those of the UK Patent Office, called *Official Journal (Patents)* (which appears weekly), and the US Patent Office, called *Official Gazette of the United States Patent and Trademark* (also weekly). Finally there is a list of seven books on patent law, all post-1978.

Incidentally it is worth noting that books on UK patenting procedures published before 1978 are obsolete as a consequence of the British Patents Act 1977 which came into effect in 1978 concurrent with the European Patent Convention and the Patent Co-operation Treaty. General enquiries concerning both British and foreign patents may be made at the Holborn Reading Rooms of the Science Reference Library in London. Finally, the journal *Vaccine* provides world-wide information on patents relevant to vaccine design and production. Twenty to twenty-five reports appear in each issue.

Tracing and locating patents *(see* bibliography entries 490, 491)

Today, searching for biomedical patents is made relatively easy thanks to the on-line availability of a number of specialist patent files. Pergamon Infoline is clearly the best source with its *Inpadoc* and *Patsearch* databases. *Inpadoc* provides access to patent documents published by 51 national and regional patent offices including those of France (1968–), Germany (1973–), Japan (1973–), the UK (1969–) and the USA (1968–). Over 10 000 000 records are on the weekly updated file (data on new documents are available within seven days of publication). *Patsearch* provides abstracts and bibliographic data for all US patents since 1971. This file is updated weekly and contains a million records.

Some abstracting services, like *Life Sciences Collection* and *Telegen,* also cover patents but of course much more selectively and long after their appearance on the above databases.

5.6 REFERENCE WORKS *(see* bibliography entries 492–496)
Guides to the literature

Today, because of the large, ever-increasing amount of available information, guides to the literature and other information services should be an indispensable tool for anyone whose job, research or study requires him or her to seek out information. In immunology this must include everyone: students, librarians, researchers, business managers in biotechnology, and so on. The larger or more complex the field (immunology is a member of both categories) or the newer one is to the field, the greater is the need to be guided through the information jungle.

The paradox is, however, that despite their importance guides are neither numerous nor popular. Part of the reason for this is that many are poorly produced, and show no understanding of the subject or the user's needs. They may have limited horizons — either they are produced by librarians for librarians, or at the very least, for the tiny body of people who are positively enthusiastic about information (rare beasts); and part rests with their failure to address themselves to the precise fields in which people actually work — one cannot expect an immunologist to identify with or find much of interest in a guide covering the entire medical sciences.

There is also one further, more serious reason: the value of being well informed about the sources of information in one's chosen field (i.e. the journals, books, organizations) is not generally recognized. Many researchers for instance still pay allegiance to the practice of serendipidity (the happy discovery of things by accident) while others consider that they have managed quite nicely to date, so why embroil themselves in activities which they care little for anyway?

The flaw in these arguments is of course that today in a subject like immunology, where research and commercial competition is fierce, technological change rapid, and government intervention in science and industry increasing, we can no longer solely rely on the fruits of accidental discovery.

There are no guides specifically covering immunology that we know of; there are, however, a number which come close.

Information sources in biotechnology, by Crafts-Lighty (1983), is the best. Monoclonal antibodies, interferon, lymphokines and vaccines are all aspects of immunology which fall into the category of biotechnology and are covered in some detail in this book. Some 70 books (mostly published between 1980 and 1983) and 26 immunology conference proceedings are listed; and approximately 30 immunology journals, plus many which are relevant but not completely immunological are included, together with brief descriptions of their subject coverage. A number of indexing and abstracting services covering immunology are also mentioned. Other chapters in the book are of interest: 'Computer databases'; 'Organisations'; and 'Patents and patenting'.

On the face of it *Information sources in the medical sciences*, edited by Morton and Godbolt (3rd edn, 1984), which is a revised and updated edition of *The use of medical literature* (edited by Morton (1977)), should be very useful. Unfortunately only nine out of the 500 pages are devoted to immunology and transplantation. Despite the newness of the work many of the comments are very dated — an eight-year-old abstracting service (*Immunological Abstracts*) is called new; a remark that the history of immunology is now attracting attention is supported by a 1971 reference. It lists 40 primary journals, including the *Mouse News Letter* but omitting many more important ones; 20 serials; and just over 40 immunological texts, mostly post-1980. The bibliographic references are inconsistent. The 2nd edition at least made an attempt to describe the periodicals, but surprisingly the descriptions have been dropped in the 3rd edition. One hopes the other chapters in the book are not written so indifferently.

Directory of cancer research information resources, by the National Cancer Institute (1979), provides cancer researchers, many of them immunologists, with a listing of most of the available cancer information sources around the world. The *Direc-*

tory is divided into 12 sections which include primary and secondary publications, classification schemes, libraries, research projects, information sources and organizations. Eight immunology journals are included with information about their publishers, frequency, classification, size, and other features. Addresses and information on organizations funding immunology are also found.

Veterinary immunology is very poorly served in *Information sources in agriculture and food science*, edited by Lilley (1981); only one book is mentioned and that (published in 1977) is out of date now.

Chen's *Health sciences information sources* is an extremely thorough and professional bibliographic guide to the medical literature. Allergy and immunology are treated separately in almost all of the book's major sections: bibliographies, dictionaries, handbooks, etc. Treatment is naturally selective, only four immunology journals being listed, for instance. Although it was published in 1981, much of the information refers to the late 1970s, therefore in a field like immunology, where growth has been both rapid and recent, the work will be found wanting. Brief annotations are provided for most items. However, for a detailed and wide view of the vast medical literature this is an excellent reference work.

Dictionaries, encyclopedias, glossaries

(*see* bibliography entries 497–514)

Such is the speed of progress in immunology that unless a textbook is updated at least every five years it suffers a severe risk of redundancy. So what role can reference works such as handbooks, encyclopedias, glossaries, compendia, and subject dictionaries have in the literature of immunology when their compilation and publication can easily take longer than five years? The simple answer is, probably very little to the worker at the forefront of immunological research; but for those requiring a grounding in immunology, reference books may at least provide a starting point.

Some immunology textbooks perform a function similar to reference works, with the advantage that the former usually are revised much more frequently. One very good example is *Basic and clinical immunology* by Stites *et al.* (1982), now in its fourth edition. It contains an appendix which includes a glossary of immunological terms and acronyms and abbreviations commonly used in immunology. This book is available in eight different languages.

Practical immunology, by Hudson and Hay (1980), contains useful information on buffers and media, equipment (with a manufacturer's index), summary tables of immunochemical data, and nomograms for ammonium sulphate solutions and for the computation of relative centrifugal forces.

Volume 3 of the *Handbook of experimental immunology*, edited by Weir (1978), has the following appendices: 1. Statistical aspects of planning and design of an immunological experiment; 2. Statistical methods as applied to immunological data; 3. Mineral oil adjuvants and the immunizing of laboratory animals; 4. Laboratory animal techniques for immunology; and 5. Mouse breeding for immunology.

The *Allergy encyclopedia*, edited by the Asthma and Allergy Foundation of America (1981), is specifically written for the patient (a rarity in the medical sciences!) and attempts to answer the most commonly occurring questions; it is good value at £4.50 (1983).

The *Compendium of immunology*, by Schwartz (1980–), covers all the important current topics in basic immunology. It is a quick-reference sourcebook and summarizes selected papers from the immunological literature. It deals with 384 topics, and provides 700 references.

The most important reference book, and compulsory reading for all immunologists and those in allied fields, is *A dictionary of immunology*, edited by Herbert *et al.* (1984), and now, thankfully, fully revised from the outdated second edition published in 1977. The third edition is some 50 pages longer, and twice as expensive, but at £7.50 still good value. Notable improvements include new entries in the fields of immunogenetics and lymphocyte nomenclature. Some old entries, not all immunological, have been dropped. This book is compiled by members of staff of various departments of Glasgow University, and of its Institute of Virology.

The appearance of the above book effectively supersedes the *Glossary of immunological terms*, by Halliday (1971), and *Glossary of hematological and serological terms*, by Samson (1973), which are both now only of historical interest.

Covering related fields, *A dictionary of virology*, edited by Rowson *et al.* (1981), and *Dictionary of microbiology*, by Singleton and Sainsbury (1981), include immunological terms — albeit relating to bacteria and viruses. *Biotechnology made simple — a glossary of recombinant DNA and hybridoma technology*, compiled and published by PJB Publications of Richmond, is an attractive aid for the non-specialist in biotechnology. Part 1 describes, in fairly simple terms, the production of monoclonal antibodies and interferon, and gives a good account of genetic engineering. Part 2 is a glossary of over 500 terms associated with biotechnology, consisting of one- to two-line explanations. Unfortunately very few will be able to afford the £75 demanded for this book, which, although nicely packaged, contains material taken directly from the pages of other texts.

The coverage of immunology by scientific encyclopedias is generally quite readable, assuming of course one can get hold of the most recent edition. The *McGraw-Hill encyclopedia of science and technology* (1982) and *Van Nostrand's scientific encyclopedia* (1983) both provide fairly reasonable introductory accounts covering approximately four pages. The ubiquitous *Encyclopaedia Britannica* (1976) contains an excellent and comprehensive section on immunology and immunity amounting to some 12 pages. It is written by J. H. Humphrey of the National Institute of Medical Research, London (hopefully there will be an update to it soon).

There are literally scores of medical dictionaries and encyclopedias containing varying amounts of immunology — usually of a clinical nature. The *Encyclopedia of clinical assessment*, edited by Woody (1980), contains over 9000 entries in its two volumes. Dictionaries like *Black's Medical dictionary* (1979) and *Butterworth's Medical dictionary* (1980) can only do limited justice to fields like immunology; probably the best of this type is *Stedman's Medical dictionary* (1983), now in its 24th edition. Of novel value is the *Inverted medical dictionary* by Rigal (1976), although it is somewhat old now, which provides 13 000 meanings reduced to key phrases, followed by the appropriate medical term — quite a feat in 267 pages.

Biographical directories (*see* bibliography entries 515–523)

Using *American Men and Women of Science* on-line on DIALOG certainly takes much of the leg work out of finding out about North American immunologists, who must themselves account for the vast bulk of the world's immunologists. Over 130 000 American and Canadian scientists actively working in the physical and biological sciences are present on the database. Through the on-line index (immunology is a descriptor term), 2806 immunologists can be located. It is also possible to search on a researcher's subject speciality (i.e. immunology of cancer, hybridoma technology). For each immunologist the following information is provided: discipline and subject specialities, personal data, education, language proficiency, professional experience, concurrent positions, memberships of societies, description of research activities, and address.

In addition to searching on discipline and subject speciality it is also possible to search on: language proficiency (e.g. all immunologists who can read Latin), honours and awards (Nobel prize winners), and the research activities field (thus a search for the term *monoclonals*, not indexed by the database, yields 52 references, all taken from this field).

Another on-line biographical file of some interest to those seeking data on outstanding American (Canadian, Mexican and US) immunologists is *Marquis Who's Who*, on DIALOG. While not as comprehensive as *American Men and Women of Science* (just 254 immunologists can be located through the on-line index), it is more current, with a quarterly updating programme, as against *American Men and Women of Science*'s three-yearly update, and it does offer different approaches to the data; you can search for women immunologists, Catholic immunologists, or members of a particular society such as the American Association of Immunologists.

Two other US publications, both in print form only, are worth mentioning: *Federation of American Societies for Experimental Biology — Directory of Members*, which covers about 20 000 scientists including all members of the American Association of Immunologists, who can be located via the society index; and *Directory of medical specialists*, a subject-arranged work which lists immunologists right at the beginning under the heading 'Allergy and immunology'.

The *International Medical Who's Who* is useful for tracing immunologists of other countries as well as the USA. With no subject index the work is only useful for tracing known immunologists. As with any international work, coverage is patchy. I. Roitt (Professor, Department of Immunology of Middlesex Hospital Medical School) is included, but not Cesar Milstein (British expert on immunoglobulins and recent Nobel Prize winner). Each entry gives, in addition to the standard biographical data, a brief abstract on medical interests. Thus the entry for Jacob Natrig, the Norwegian immunologist, provides the following details: 'immunology research, particularly human immuno-globulin structure, genetic markers and human lymphocyte markers; immunology, rheumatoid inflammation and amyloidosis'.

5.7 AUDIOVISUAL AIDS

The enterprising American Society of Clinical Pathologists (ASCP) has produced a variety of audiovisual aids in the field of clinical immunology. They are mainly 25–35 minute video-cassettes with supplementary material, available from Raven Press. Titles include:

Basic concepts in immunology (1978)

Cellular immunity and immune deficiency diseases (1981)

Diagnostic evaluation of auto-immune diseases (1979)

Mechanisms of auto-immune diseases

Mechanisms of immunologic tissue injury (1978)

T- and B-lymphocytes: their identification in peripheral blood and solid tissue
(1978)

The cassettes are priced at $374 (1983 prices), which works out at about $12 a
minute!

Also obtainable from Raven Press is a set of 131 ASCP 35 mm slides entitled
Atlas of autoimmune diseases (1976) and costing $129.20 (1983 prices).

5.8 LIBRARY CLASSIFICATION SCHEMES AS APPLIED TO IMMUNOLOGY (*see* bibliography entries 524–529)

In a survey on the information needs of virologists (*Virology: an information profile,*
London: Mansell, 1983), we concluded that while virologists generally liked
reading the virological and scientific literature, few actually enjoyed the process
of searching libraries or examining bibliographies and abstracting and indexing
services — although they all appeared to do it regularly.

It cannot be a generalization to say that the same must be true for immunologists (and the scientific community come to that) for finding out where a book,
periodical, proceedings or report is located in a library, catalogue or bibliography
can prove to be a nightmare.

Why is this? Part of the blame can be laid at the feet of the numerous classification schemes in existence; none of them was designed to cope with the huge
expansion in the quantity and diversity seen in the biomedical literature over the
last 20–30 years. Little agreement exists as to precisely what particular subject
arrangement would be most useful. In a field such as immunology there are a
number of user groups — immunologists, microbiologists, biochemists, medical
practitioners, veterinary scientists and many others — who all view the field
from fundamentally different stances; and all those viewpoints translate into
quite different classification schemes for ordering documents on shelves or in
bibliographies.

Table 5.6   Classification schemes in use in UK libraries

	Used by (%)	Total numbers
Own scheme	33	(122)
NLM	14.9	(55)
Barnard	14	(52)
UDC	13.8	(51)
Dewey	13.5	(50)
LC	5.4	(20)
Bliss	3	(11)
Others — Boston, MRC, Garside, Bodleian — less than 1% each		

Based on an examination of 370 specialist libraries
in the UK.

Table 5.7   *Different approaches to classifying books*

Book	Dewey	LC	Bliss	Barnard
Antibody as a tool. The applications of immunochemistry (Marchalonis and Warr, 1982)	574.2′9	QR 183.6	HPG BP	HB.AT.MAR
Practical immunology (Hudson and Hay, 1980)	574.2′9	QR 181	HPH	HB.HUD
Parasitic diseases: Vol. 1, *Immunology* (Mansfield, 1981)	616.9′6	RC 119	HRI FLS	LH.MAN
Clinical aspects of immunology (Lachmann and Peters, 1982)	616.07′9	QR 181	HSU	HB.O.GEL
General immunology (Cooper, 1982)	574.2′9	QR 181	HPG	HB.COO

Table 5.8   *The location of immunology in the Barnard Classification*

Location	Subject
G	Toxicology and diseases of chemical causation
H	Immunology and infectious diseases
HA	Infection
HB	Immunity
HG	Serology
HI	Immunization
HW	Infectious diseases in general
J	Bacteriology
K	Virology and Viral Diseases
P	Pathology (tumour viruses)
Q	Diagnosis and Clinical Medicine
RK–RV	Therapeutics, etc.
X	Veterinary Science

A further complication in immunology is that it has only recently emerged as a subject in its own right. Consequently much of its literature still resides in other areas such as medicine, microbiology, pathology, etc.

The problems that arise from attempting to classify biomedical documents can best be illustrated by the fact that of 370 specialist medical libraries in the UK, about a third have had to devise their own tailor-made classification schemes (*Table 5.6*).

Table 5.9 *The location of immunology in the Bliss classification scheme*

Location	Subject
HP	DISEASES AND PATHOLOGY
HPG	Immune reaction, immunology, immunity
HPH	Antigens and antibodies
HPI	Antibodies
HPJ	Types of antibody
HPJ L	Types of immunity
HSU	Immunologic diseases, immunopathology
HSV	Hypersensitivity, allergies
HSV X	Autoimmune disease
HSX	Anatomical and physiological disorders

Table 5.10 *The location of immunology in the Dewey Decimal classification*

Location	Subject
574	BIOLOGY
. 2	Pathology
. 29	Immunity (class here autoimmunity, immunology, immunogenetics)
.292	Antigens
.293	Antibodies
.295	Immune reaction
591	ZOOLOGY
. 2	Pathology
. 23–29	Causes and immunity
616	DISEASES
.079	Immunity (immunology); class here autoimmunity, immunogenetics
612	HUMAN PHYSIOLOGY
. 11	Blood
.118.22	Immunity (immunology)

The other main schemes likely to be encountered are that of the National Library of Medicine (NLM), Barnard, the Universal Decimal Classification (UDC), Dewey, the Library of Congress (LC) scheme and Bliss; all have their disadvantages. Only Barnard (1955) and NLM (1979) have had the foresight to

Table 5.11   The location of immunology in the Library of Congress classification scheme

Notation	Subject
Q	SCIENCE
QR	Microbiology
QR 46	Medical microbiology
QR 49	Veterinary microbiology
65	Techniques
180	Immunology
184	Immunogenetics
185	Types of immunity
186	Immune response
187	General works
188	Hypersensitivity. Allergy
.3	Autoimmunity
.4	Tolerance
.5	Radiation immunology
.6	Tumour immunology
.8	Transplantation immunology
189	Vaccines — by disease A–Z
201	Pathogenic organisms A–Z
355	Virology
R	MEDICINE
RA 638	Public health
RM 270–282	Serum therapy
S	AGRICULTURE
SF	Veterinary science
757.2	Veterinary immunology
781	Virus diseases of animals

provide immunology with its own class designation: H — Immunology and Infectious Diseases (Barnard); and QW — Microbiology and Immunology (NLM). With Barnard, the bulk of immunology will be found between HB and HI; inevitably aspects of microbial immunity will be located under J — Bacteriology and K — Virology. Because it has been more recently revised, NLM uses more modern terminology than Barnard; immunological documents will be found chiefly between QW 500 and QW 949. NLM's scheme will also be met when searching *Medline*, the giant computer abstracting service.

Table 5.12 The location of immunology in the National Library of Medicine's classification scheme

Location	Subject
QV	PHARMACOLOGY
QW	MICROBIOLOGY AND IMMUNOLOGY
1	Societies
4	General works
25	Laboratory manuals
70	Veterinary microbiology
160	Viruses (general), virology
500	IMMUNOLOGY
700	Infection, mechanism of infection and resistance
730	Virulence
800	Biological products producing immunity
805	Vaccines, etc.
806	Vaccination
815	Immune serums
949	Vaccine therapy
WC	INFECTIOUS DISEASES
QZ	PATHOLOGY

Unlike Barnard and NLM, LC (1973) attempts to cover the entire field of knowledge and this it does by using a mixed notation of letters and numbers. Immunological documents are mainly found, subsumed under Microbiology, between QR 180 and QR 189, with Serum Therapy at RM 270–282 and Veterinary Immunology at SF 757.2.

Bliss (1980) is a modern scheme which uses modern terminology. However it effectively splits immunology into two parts: the bulk under Diseases and Pathology at HPG–HPJ; and the remainder under Clinical Aspects at HSU–HSV. Its 'faceted' structure however enables a degree of specification unique among classification schemes.

Dewey is probably the most widely encountered classification scheme in public libraries. It was laid down over a century ago and has undergone revisions in an effort to cope with the literature explosion. Unfortunately immunology has not fared too well; Dewey provides the librarian with an opportunity to scatter it to the four corners of the biological sciences: Pathology, Zoology, Diseases and Human Physiology. In practice most librarians plump for 574.27, under Pathology.

Similar problems will be found in the UDC scheme, Immunology being located at 57.083 (techniques); 575 (genetics); 577.27 (molecular immunology), and 612.017 (immunity).

Table 5.13 The location of immunology in the Universal Decimal System (UDC)

Location	Subject
57	BIOLOGICAL SCIENCES IN GENERAL. VIROLOGY. MICROBIOLOGY
57.083	Microbiological, virological and immunological methods and techniques
.083. 2 } .083.36 }	Immunological methods, reaction
575	GENERAL GENETICS. GENERAL CYTOGENETICS. IMMUNOGENETICS. EVOLUTION. SPECIATION. PHYLOGENY.
577	MATERIAL. BASES OF LIFE. BIOCHEMISTRY. MOLE-CULAR BIOLOGY. BIOPHYSICS.
.27	Molecular bases of immunity. Molecular immunology
612	PHYSIOLOGY
.017. 1	Immunity
.11	Natural and inherited
.12	Artificial
. 3	Anaphylaxis. Hypersensitivity
. 4	Toxins — Antitoxins

Outlines of the main schemes seen from an immunological standpoint are shown in *Tables 5.7–5.13*.

Part II

BIBLIOGRAPHY

BIBLIOGRAPHY

ORGANIZATIONS

Directories of Organizations and Research
(*see* section 2.2)

1 *Agricultural research centres.* 7th edn. Harlow, Essex: Longman, 1983. ISBN 0-582-90014-X.

1a *Aslib directory of information sources in the United Kingdom.* 5th edn. London. Aslib, 1982. ISBN 0-85124-166-0.

1b *Commercial biotechnology: an international analysis.* Washington, D.C.: US Congressional Office of Technology Assessment, 1984.

2 Department of Health and Social Security. *DHSS Handbook of Research and Development.* London: HMSO, annual.

2a *Biotechnology Newswatch.* New York: McGraw-Hill, 1983.

3 *Directory of British Associations.* Beckenham, Kent: CBD Research, 1965–. Irregular. ISSN 0070-5152.

4 *Directory of European Associations.* Beckenham, Kent: CBD Research, 1971–. Irregular. Pt. 1, ISSN 0070-5500: Pt. 2, ISSN 0309-5339.

5 *Directory of grant-making trusts.* Tonbridge, Kent: Charities Aid Foundation. Annual. ISBN 0-904757-15-3.

6 *Directory of Health Science Libraries in the United States.* Cleveland, Ohio: Baxter School of Library Science, 1969–. Irregular. ISSN 0095-7925.

6a *Directory of medical specialists.* 19th edn. Chicago: Marquis, 1979. ISBN 0-8379-0519-2.

7 *Encyclopedia of medical organizations and agencies.* Detroit: Gale, 1983. ISBN 0-8103-0347-7.

8 *European research centres.* 5th edn. Harlow, Essex: Longman, 1983. ISBN 0-582-90012-3.

9 *Federal Research in Progress.* Springfield, Virginia: National Technical Information Service (currently initiated projects and those recently completed). *Host:* DIALOG.

10 *Foundation Directory.* New York: The Foundation Center. Semi-annual updates. *Host:* DIALOG.

11   *Foundation Grants Index.* New York: The Foundation Center, 1973–. Bimonthly updates. *Host:* DIALOG.

11a *Genetic Engineering and Biotechnology Yearbook 1983.* New York: Elsevier, 1983.

12   *Grants.* Phoenix, Arizona: Oryx Press, 1977–. Monthly updates. *Host:* DIALOG.

13   *The Grants Register.* London: Macmillan, 1969–. Biennial. ISSN 0072-5471.

13a *The guide to corporate-sponsored university research in biotechnology.* New York: Genetic Sciences International, 1983.

14   *Industrial research in the United Kingdom: a guide to organizations and programmes.* 10th edn. Harlow, Essex: Longman, 1983. ISBN 0-582-90016-6.

15   *International biotechnology directory: products, companies, research and organizations.* New York: Macmillan, 1983. ISBN 0-333-35140-1.

16   *International Research Centers Directory.* Detroit: Gale, 1982 (3 issues). Irregular. ISSN 0278-2731.

17   *Medical and Health Information Directory.* Detroit: Gale, 1978–. Triennial.

18   *Medical research centres.* 6th edn. Harlow, Essex: Longman, 1984. ISBN 0-582-90017-4.

19   *Medical Research Council Handbook 1970–76.* London: Medical Research Council, 1977. ISSN 0309-1032.

20   *The medical research directory.* Chichester, Sussex: John Wiley, 1983. ISBN 0-471-10335-7.

21   *Medical research index.* 5th edn. Harlow, Essex: Longman, 1979. ISBN 0-587-90005-0.

21a *The New Biotechnology Market Place: The Telegen Directory of Japanese Biotechnology.* New York: EIC/Intelligence, 1983.

22   *National Biomedical Research Directory.* Bethesda, Maryland: National Health Directory, 1980.

23   *New Research Centres.* Detroit: Gale, 1965–. Thrice yearly. ISSN 0028-6591.

24   *Research Centers Directory.* Detroit: Gale, 1960–. Irregular. ISSN 0090–1518.

25   *Research Awards Index.* US National Institutes of Health. Washington, D.C.: US Government Printing Office, 1949–. Annual. ISSN 0147-5320.

26   *Research in British Universities, Polytechnics and Colleges:* Volume 2, *Biological Sciences.* Boston Spa, West Yorkshire: British Library Lending Division, 1980–. Annual. ISSN 0143-0734.

27   *SSIE Current Research.* Springfield, Virginia: National Technical Information Service, 1978–82. *Host:* DIALOG.

27a *The Telegen Directory of US Biotechnology.* New York: EIC/Intelligence, 1983.

28   *Trade Associations and Professional Bodies of the United Kingdom.* Oxford: Pergamon Press, 1967–. Irregular. ISSN 0082-5689.

28a *World guide to scientific associations and learned societies*. 4th edn. Munich: K.G. Saur, 1984. ISBN 3-598-20522-8.

29   *World guide to special libraries*. Munich: K.G. Saur, 1983. ISBN 3-598-20528-7.

30   *World of Learning*. London: Europa, 1947–. Annual. ISSN 0084-2117.

31   *Yearbook of International Organizations*. Brussels: Union of International Associations, 1949–. Biennial. ISSN 0084-3814.

CONFERENCES

Lists of Forthcoming Conferences *(see* section 4.2)

32   *Forthcoming International Scientific and Technical Conferences*. London: Aslib, 1951–. Quarterly. ISSN 0046-4686.

33   *World Meetings: Outside the United States and Canada*. Chestnut Hill, New York: Macmillan, 1968–. Quarterly. ISSN 0043-8677.

34   *World Meetings: United States and Canada*. Chestnut Hill, New York: Macmillan, 1963–. Quarterly. ISSN 0043–8693.

Directories of Conference Proceedings *(see* section 4.3)

35   *Conference Papers Index*. Riverdale, Maryland: Cambridge Scientific Abstracts, 1977–. Monthly. ISSN 0162–704X.

36   *Directory of Published Proceedings. Series SEMT (Science, Engineering, Medicine and Technology)*. Harrison, New York: Interdok, 1965–. 10 p.a. ISSN 0012-3293.

37   *Index of Conference Proceedings Received by the BLL*. Boston Spa, West Yorkshire, UK: British Library Lending Division, 1964–. Monthly. ISSN 0305-5183.

38   *Index to Scientific and Technical Proceedings*. Philadelphia: Institute for Scientific Information, 1978–. Monthly. ISSN 0149-8088.

39   *Proceedings in Print*. Arlington, Massachusetts: Proceedings in Print Inc., 1964–. Bimonthly. ISSN 0032-9568.

40   *System for Information on Grey Literature in Europe*. Munich: Inka, 1981. Bimonthly updates.

Major Conferences *(see* section 4.4)

41   British Society for Immunology Meetings. 1955–. 3/4 a year.

42   Collegium Internationale Allergologicum Symposia. 1954–. Biennial.

43   European Academy of Allergy and Clinical Immunology Congresses. 1971–. Annual.

44 Federation of American Societies for Experimental Biology Symposia. 1916–. Annual.

45 Hybridoma Research Congresses. 1982–. Annual.

46 ICN-UCLA Symposia on Molecular Biology. 1972–. Approx. 2 a year.

47 International Association of Biological Standardization Congresses, Symposia and Meetings. 1954–. Congresses: every two years; Symposia: 2 per year; Meetings: annual.

48 International Congresses of Immunology. 1971–. Triennial.

49 International Convocations on Immunology. 1968–. Approx. biennial.

50 International Symposia on Immunopathology. 1959–. Approx. biennial.

51 International Union of Immunological Societies Symposia. 1971–. Approx. annual.

52 National Reticulo-endothelial Society Meetings. 1963–. Annual.

53 Royal Society of Medicine Meetings. 1834–. 3/4 a year.

54 Transplantation Society Congresses. 1966–. Biennial.

Proceedings (*see* section 4.6)

55 *Developments in Biological Standardization*. Geneva: S. Karger for the International Association of Biological Standardization. 1955–. 2/3 a year. ISSN 0301-5149.

56 *Developments in Immunology*. Amsterdam: Elsevier, 1978–. 3/4 a year.

57 *ICN-UCLA Symposia on Molecular Biology*. New York: Academic Press, 1971–. 2 a year.

58 *Immunopathology*. New York: Grune & Stratton, 1959–. Approx. every 2 years. ISSN 0073–5531.

59 *INSERM Symposia*. Amsterdam: Elsevier, 1971–. Approx. 2 a year.

60 *International Congress series*. Amsterdam: Elsevier, 1969–. As many as 4/5 a year.

61 *International Convocations on Immunology*. Basel: S. Karger, 1969–. Approx. every 2 years. ISSN 0074-4220.

62 *Menarini Series on Immunopathology*. New York: Springer Verlag, 1979–. Irregular.

63 *Perspectives in Immunology*. New York: Academic Press, 1969–. Irregular.

64 *Progress in Immunology*. New York: Academic Press, 1969–. Approx. biennial.

65 *Symposia Fondation Merieux*. Amsterdam: Elsevier, 1979–. 3/4 a year.

66 *Symposia of the Giovanni Lorenzini Foundation*. Amsterdam: Elsevier, 1975–. 2/3 a year.

67 *Transplantation Today*. New York: Grune & Stratton, 1967–. Biennial. ISSN 0074-3984.

IMMUNOLOGY: ITS LITERATURE

Lists of Journals (*see* section 5.1)

68 *British Union Catalogue of Periodicals (BUCOP)*. London: Butterworths, 1955–1981. Quarterly.

69 *Canadian Locations of Journals Indexed for Medline*. Ottawa: National Research Council, 1970–. Annual. ISSN 0070-7629.

70 *Conser Microfiche*. Ottawa: National Library of Canada. Annual.

71 *Current Serials Received*. Boston Spa, West Yorkshire: British Library Lending Division, 1965–. Annual. ISSN 0309-0655.

72 *Health Sciences Serials*. Bethesda, Maryland: National Library of Medicine, 1979–. Quarterly. (Microfiche only.) ISSN 0162-0843.

73 *Index to NLM Serial Titles*. Bethesda, Maryland: National Library of Medicine, 1981. 4th edn.

74 *Irregular Serials and Annuals*. New York: Bowker, 1967–. Biennial. ISSN 0000-0043.

75 *ISDS Register*. Paris: International Serials Data System International Centre. Bimonthly. (Microfiche only.)

76 *Keyword Index to Serial Titles*. Boston Spa, West Yorkshire: British Library Lending Division, 1979–. Updated quarterly. (Microfiche only.)

77 *List of Journals Abstracted by Excerpta Medica*. Amsterdam: Elsevier Science Division, 1964–. ISSN 0167-6180.

78 *List of Journals Abstracted by Life Sciences Collection*. Bethesda, Maryland: Cambridge Scientific Abstracts, 1983.

79 *List of Journals Indexed in Index Medicus*. Bethesda, Maryland: National Library of Medicine, 1960–. ISSN 0093-3821.

80 *List of Serials Indexed for Online Users*. Bethesda, Maryland: National Library of Medicine, 1980–. ISSN 0736-7139.

81 *Medical Serials and Books in Print*. New York: Bowker. Annual.

82 *List Bio-med: Biomedical Serials in Scandinavian Libraries*. Gothenburg: Universitetsbiblioteket, 1965–. ISSN 0075-9813.

83 *New Serial Titles*. Washington, DC: Library of Congress, 1953–. Monthly. ISSN 0028-6680.

84 *New Serial Titles — Classed Subject Arrangement*. Washington, D.C.: Library of Congress, 1955–80. Monthly. ISSN 0028-6699.

85 *Periodicals Held by the Science Reference Library*.

86 OCLC. Columbus, Ohio: OCLC.

87 *Periodicals relevant to microbiology and immunology*. Marseille: International Union of Microbiological Societies, 1968.

88   *Serial Sources for BIOSIS Database.* Philadelphia: Biosciences Information Service, 1970–. Annual. ISSN 0067-8937.

89   *Serials in the British Library.* London: British Library, 1981–. Quarterly. ISSN 0260-005.

90   *Serline.* Bethesda, Maryland: National Library of Medicine. Monthly updates. *Host:* BLAISE-Link.

91   *Ulrich's International Periodical Directory.* New York: Bowker, 1932–. Annual. ISSN 0000-0175.

92   *Ulrich's Quarterly.* New York: Bowker, 1977–. Quarterly. ISSN 0000-0507.

93   **University of London.** *Union List of Serials.* 1977–. Semi-annual.

Indexing, Abstracting and Current-Awareness Services (*see* section 5.1)

94   *BioEssays.* Cambridge: Cambridge University Press. 1984–. Monthly. ISSN 0265-9247.

94a   *Biological Abstracts.* Philadelphia: Bioscience Information Service, 1927–. Semi-monthly. ISSN 0192-6935.

95   *Biological Abstracts/RRM.* Philadelphia: Bioscience Information Service, 1965–. Semi-monthly. ISSN 0192-6985.

96   *Bioresearch Today: Cancer C — Immunology.* Philadelphia: Bioscience Information Service, 1972–. Monthly. ISSN 0149-1032.

97   *Bioscope.* Sheffield: Biomedical Information Service, University of Sheffield, 1984–. Monthly.

98   *Biosis/CAC Selects.* Philadelphia: Bioscience Information Service, 1980–. Monthly.

99   *Biotechnology Abstracts.* The Hague: Martinus Nijhoff, 1982–. Monthly.

100   *Bulletin Signalétique:* Part 340, *Microbiologie–Virologie–Immunologie.* Paris: Centre National de la Recherche Scientifique, 1961–. Monthly. ISSN 0007-5450.

101   *Bulletin Signalétique:* Part 251, *Cancernet/Cancerologie, Oncology.* Paris: Centre National de la Recherche Scientifique, 1969–. Monthly. ISSN 0245-9566.

101a *Current Advances in Immunology.* Oxford: Pergamon Press, 1984–. Monthly. ISSN 0741-1650.

102   *Current Awareness in the Biological Sciences.* Oxford: Pergamon Press, 1956–. Monthly. ISSN 0733-4443.

103   *Current Contents/Life Sciences.* Philadelphia: Institute for Scientific Information, 1958–. Weekly. ISSN 0011-3409.

104   *Current Contents/Agriculture, Biology and Environmental Sciences.* Philadelphia: Institute for Scientific Information, 1970–. Weekly. ISSN 0090-0508.

105   *Current Titles in Immunology, Transplantation and Allergy.* London: Msk Books, 1980–. Semi-monthly. ISSN 0301-0007.

106   *Economy Bulletins*. Sheffield: Biomedical Information Service, University of Sheffield, 1970–. Monthly. ISSN (various).

107   *Excerpta Medica:* Section 26, *Immunology, Serology and Transplantation*. Amsterdam: Elsevier Science Publishers, 1946–. Monthly. ISSN 0014-4304.

108   *Express Bulletins*. Sheffield: Biomedical Information Service, University of Sheffield, 1970–. Monthly. ISSN (various).

109   *ICRDB Cancergrams*. Bethesda, Maryland: US National Cancer Institute, 1978–. Monthly. ISSN (various).

110   *Immunization: Abstracts and Bibliography*. Atlanta, Georgia: Center for Disease Control, 1979–. Thrice-yearly. ISSN 0196-4917.

111   *Immunology Abstracts*. Bethesda, Maryland: Cambridge Scientific Abstracts, 1976–. Monthly. ISSN 0307-112X.

112   *Index Medicus*. Bethesda, Maryland: National Library of Medicine, 1960–. Monthly. ISSN 0019-3879.

113   *Index Veterinarius*. Slough, Berkshire: Commonwealth Agricultural Bureaux, 1933–. Monthly. ISSN 0019-6438.

114   *International Pharmaceutical Abstracts*. Bethesda, Maryland: American Society of Hospital Pharmacists, 1964–. Semi-monthly. ISSN 0020-8264.

115   *Promt*. Cleveland, Ohio: Predicasts, 1972–. Weekly.

116   *Science Citation Index*. Philadelphia: Institute for Scientific Information, 1961–. Bimonthly. ISSN 0036-827X.

117   *Telegen Reporter*. New York: EIC/Intelligence, 1982–. Monthly.

118   *Veterinary Bulletin*. Slough, Berkshire: Commonwealth Agricultural Bureaux, 1931–. Monthly. ISSN 0042-4854.

119   *Zentralblatt für Bakteriologie, Mikrobiologie und Hygiene* ('Abstracts of Microbiology and Hygiene'): 1. Abt., *Referate Abstracts*. Berne: Gustav Fischer Verlag, 1879–. Monthly. ISSN 0044-4073.

On-line Databases Covering Journal Articles
(*see* section 5.1)

120   *BIOSIS/BIOSIS Previews*. Philadelphia: Biosciences Information Service, 1969–. Weekly updates. *Hosts:* BRS, Data-Star, DIALOG, Dimdi, ESA-IRS, Orbit.

121   *Biotechnology*. London: Derwent Publications, 1982–. Monthly updates. *Host:* Orbit.

122   *CAB Abstracts*. Slough, Berkshire: Commonwealth Agricultural Bureaux, 1972–. Monthly updates. *Hosts:* DIALOG, Dimdi, ESA-IRS.

123   *Cancernet*. Bethesda, Maryland: National Library of Medicine, 1967–. Monthly updates. *Hosts:* BLAISE-Link, Dimdi.

124 *Cancernet.* Paris: CNRS, 1968–. Monthly updates. *Host:* Télésystèmes-Questel.

125 *Current Awareness in the Biological Sciences.* London: Pergamon, 1983–. Monthly updates. *Host:* Pergamon-Infoline.

126 *Embase.* Amsterdam: Elsevier, 1974–. Monthly updates. *Hosts:* Data-Star, DIALOG, Dimdi.

127 *International Pharmaceutical Abstracts.* Bethesda: American Association of Hospital Pharmacists, 1970–. Monthly updates. *Hosts:* BRS, DIALOG.

128 *IRC Medical Science.* Amsterdam: Elsevier, 1982–. Twice-monthly updates. *Host:* BRS.

129 *Life Sciences Collection.* Bethesda, Maryland: Cambridge Scientific Abstracts, 1978–. Monthly updates. *Host:* DIALOG.

130 *Medline.* Bethesda, Maryland: National Library of Medicine, 1964–. Monthly updates. *Hosts:* BLAISE-Link, BRS, Data-Star, DIALOG, Dimdi, NLM.

131 *Pre-med.* New York: BRS. Latest 3–4 months. Weekly updates. *Hosts:* BRS, Data-Star.

132 *PTS Promt.* Cleveland, Ohio: Predicasts Inc., 1972–. Weekly updates. *Hosts:* Data-Star, DIALOG.

133 *Scisearch.* Philadelphia: Institute for Scientific Information, 1974–. Monthly updates. *Hosts:* DIALOG, Dimdi.

134 *Telegenline.* New York: EIC Intelligence, 1973–. Monthly updates. *Hosts:* DIALOG, Dimdi, ESA-IRS.

Immunology Journals (*see* section 5.1)

135 *Acta Pathologica, Microbiologica et Immunologica Scandinavica. C Immunology* (formerly *Acta Pathologica et Microbiologica Scandinavica. Section C Immunology*). Copenhagen: Munksgaard, 1975–. Bimonthly. ISSN 0304-1328.

136 *Allergie et Immunologie.* Paris: Nouvelles Editions Médicales Françaises, 1969–. Quarterly.

137 *Allergie und Immunologie (Leipzig)* (formerly *Allergie und Asthma*). Leipzig: Johann Amrosius Barth Verlag, 1955–. Quarterly. ISSN 0002-5755.

138 *Allergologia et Immunopathologia.* Madrid: Sociedad Española de Allergía, 1972–. Bimonthly. ISSN 0301-0546.

139 *Allergologie.* Deisenhofen: Verlag Dr Karl Feistle, 1978–. Semi-monthly. ISSN 0344-5062.

140 *Allergy* (formerly *Acta Allergologica*). Copenhagen: Munksgaard, 1948–. 8 issues/yr. ISSN 0105-4358.

141 *American Journal of Reproductive Immunology.* New York: Alan R. Liss, 1980–. Bimonthly. ISSN 0271-7352.

142   *American Journal of Veterinary Research.* Schaumberg, Illinois: American Veterinary Medical Association, 1940–. Monthly. ISSN 0002-9645.

143   *Annales d'Immunologie* (formerly *Annales de l'Institut Pasteur* and *Revue d'Immunologie*). Paris: Masson, 1973–. Bimonthly. ISSN 0300-4910.

144   *Annals of Allergy.* Minneapolis: American College of Allergists, 1943–. Monthly. ISSN 0003-4738.

145   *Archivum Immunologiae et Therapiae Experimentalis (Warszawa).* Wrocław: Publishing House of the Polish Academy of Science, 1953–. Bimonthly. ISSN 0004-069X.

146   *Arthritis and Rheumatism.* Atlanta: Arthritis Foundation, 1958–. Monthly. ISSN 0004–3591.

146a   *BioTechnology.* Basingstoke: Macmillan Journals Ltd, 1983. Monthly.

147   *Blood.* New York: Grune & Stratton, 1946–. Monthly. ISSN 0006-4971.

148   *Cancer Immunology and Immunotherapy.* New York: Springer Verlag, 1976–. 6 issues/yr. ISSN 0340-7004.

149   *Cancer Research.* Baltimore: American Association for Cancer Research, 1941–. Monthly. ISSN 0008-5472.

150   *Cell.* Cambridge, Massachusetts: MIT Press, 1974–. Monthly. ISSN 0092-8674.

151   *Cellular Immunology.* New York: Academic Press, 1970–. 18 times/yr. ISSN 0008-8749.

152   *Chinese Journal of Microbiology and Immunology.* Taiwan: Chinese Society of Microbiology (co-sponsor Chinese Society of Immunology), 1968–. Quarterly. ISSN 0009-4587.

153   *Clinical Allergy.* Oxford: Blackwell Scientific Publications, for the British Society for Allergy and Clinical Immunology, 1971–. Bimonthly. ISSN 0009-9090.

154   *Clinical Chemistry.* Winston-Salem, North Carolina: American Association for Clinical Chemistry, 1955–. Monthly. ISSN 0009-9147.

155   *Clinical and Experimental Immunology.* Oxford: Blackwell Scientific Publications, for the British Society for Immunology, 1966–. Monthly. ISSN 0009-9104.

156   *Clinical Immunology and Immunopathology.* New York: Academic Press, 1972–. Monthly. ISSN 0090-1229.

157   *Clinical Immunology Newsletter.* New York: Elsevier, 1980–. Semi-monthly. ISSN 0197-1859.

158   *Clinical Immunology Reviews.* New York: Marcel Dekker, 1982–. Quarterly. ISSN 0277-9366.

159   *Clinical Reviews in Allergy.* New York: Elsevier, 1983–. Quarterly. ISSN 0731-8235.

160   *Comparative Immunology, Microbiology and Infectious Diseases*. Oxford: Pergamon Press, 1978–. Quarterly. ISSN 0147-9571.

161   *Complement*. Basel: S. Karger, 1984–. Quarterly. ISSN 0253-5076.

162   *CRC Critical Reviews in Immunology*. Boca Raton, Florida: CRC Press, 1979–. Quarterly. ISSN 0197-3355.

163   *Developmental and Comparative Immunology*. Oxford: Pergamon Press, 1977–. Quarterly. ISSN 0145-305X.

164   *Diagnostic Immunology*. Washington, D.C.: Alan R. Liss, 1983–. Quarterly. ISSN 0735-3111.

165   *European Journal of Immunology*. Weinheim: Verlag Chemie GmbH, 1970–. Monthly. ISSN 0014-2980.

165a *Experimental and Clinical Immunogenetics*. Basel: S. Karger, 1984–. Quarterly. ISSN 0254-9670.

166   *Experimental Cell Biology*. Basel: S. Karger, 1938–. Bimonthly. ISSN 0304-3568.

167   *Federation Proceedings*. Bethesda, Maryland: Federation of American Societies for Experimental Biology, 1941–. Monthly. ISSN 0014-9446.

168   *Folia Allergologica et Immunologica Clinica*. Rome: Società Italiana di Allergologia e Immunologia Clinica, 1953–. Bimonthly. ISSN 0303-8432.

169   *Frontiers in Immunoassay*. Anaheim, California: Scientific Newsletters, 1980–. Monthly. ISSN 0270-0476.

170   *Human Immunology*. New York: Elsevier, for the American Association of Clinical Histocompatibility Testing, 1980–. Quarterly. ISSN 0198-8859.

171   *Human Lymphocyte Differentiation*. Eastbourne: W. B. Saunders, 1981–. Quarterly. ISSN 0144-3909.

172   *Hybridoma*. New York: Mary Ann Liebert, 1981–. Quarterly. ISSN 0272-457X.

173   *Immunität und Infektion*. Baden-Baden, Federal Republic of Germany: Verlag Gerhard Witzstrock, 1973–. Bimonthly. ISSN 0340-1162.

174   *Immunobiology (Stuttgart) Zeitschrift für Immunitätsforschung*. Stuttgart: Gustav Fischer Verlag, 1909–. Monthly. ISSN 0340-904X.

175   *Immunogenetics*. New York: Springer Verlag, 1974–. Monthly. ISSN 0093-7711.

176   *Immunologia Polska* (formerly *Annals of Immunology*). Warsaw: Poznanskie Towarzystwo Przyjaciol Nauk — Société des Amis des Sciences et des Lettres de Poznan, 1969–. Quarterly. ISSN 0044-8338.

177   *Immunological Communications*. New York: Marcel Dekker, 1972–. Bimonthly. ISSN 0090-0877.

178   *Immunologiya* (*see also Soviet Immunology*). Moscow: Izdatel'stvo Meditsina, 1980–. Bimonthly. ISSN 0206-4952.

179 *Immunology.* Oxford: Blackwell Scientific Publications, for the British Society for Immunology, 1958–. Monthly. ISSN 0019-2805.

180 *Immunology Letters.* Amsterdam: Elsevier, for the Federation of European Immunological Societies. 1979–. Bimonthly. ISSN 0165-2478.

181 *Immunology Today.* Amsterdam: Elsevier, 1980–. Monthly. ISSN 0167-4919.

182 *Immunology Tribune.* Houston: MDT Publications, 1979–. Monthly. ISSN 0271-3284.

183 *Immunopharmacology.* New York: Elsevier, 1978–. Quarterly. ISSN 0162-3109.

184 *Infection and Immunity.* Washington, D.C.: American Society for Micro-biology, 1970–. Monthly. ISSN 0019-9567.

185 *Inflammation.* New York: Plenum Press, 1975–. Quarterly. ISSN 0360-3997.

186 *International Archives of Allergy and Applied Immunology.* Basel: S. Karger, 1950–. Monthly. ISSN 0200-5915.

187 International Journal of Cancer. Geneva: International Union against Cancer, 1966–. Monthly. ISSN 0200-7136.

188 *International Journal of Immunopharmacology.* New York: Pergamon Press, 1979–. Bimonthly. ISSN 0192-0561.

189 *IRCS Medical Science: Immunology and Allergy.* Lancaster: Elsevier-IRCS Ltd, 1973. Monthly. ISSN 0305-666X.

190 *Journal of Allergy and Clinical Immunology.* St Louis: C. V. Mosby, 1929–. Monthly. ISSN 0091-6749.

191 *Journal of Biological Response Modifiers.* New York: Raven Press, 1983. 6 per year. ISSN 0732-6580.

192 *Journal of Clinical Immunoassay.* Wayne, Michigan: Clinical Ligand Assay Society, 1978–. Quarterly. ISSN 0736-4393.

193 *Journal of Clinical Immunology.* New York: Plenum Press, 1981–. Quarterly. ISSN 0271-9142.

194 *Journal of Clinical Investigation.* New York: Rockefeller University Press, for the American Society for Clinical Investigation, 1924–. Monthly. ISSN 0021-9738.

195 *Journal of Clinical and Laboratory Immunology.* Edinburgh: Teviot Science Publishers, 1978–. Bimonthly. ISSN 0141-2760.

196 *Journal of Experimental Medicine.* New York: Rockefeller University Press, 1896–. Monthly. ISSN 0022-1007.

197 *Journal of Immunoassay.* New York: Marcel Dekker, 1980–. Quarterly. ISSN 0197-1522.

198 *Journal of Immunogenetics.* Oxford: Blackwell Scientific Publications, 1974–. Bimonthly. ISSN 0305-1811.

199 *Journal of Immunological Methods.* Amsterdam: Elsevier, 1971–. Semi-monthly. ISSN 0022-1759.

200   *Journal of Immunology*. Baltimore: Williams & Wilkins, for the American Association of Immunologists, 1916–. Monthly. ISSN 0022-1767.

201   *Journal of Immunopharmacology*. New York: Marcel Dekker, 1979–. Quarterly. ISSN 0163-0571.

202   *Journal of Infectious Diseases*. Chicago: University of Chicago, 1904–. Monthly. ISSN 0022-1899.

202a *Journal of Leukocyte Biology* (formerly *RES — The Journal of the Reticuloendothelial Society*). New York: Alan R. Liss, 1967–. ISSN 0741-5400.

203   *Journal of Molecular and Cellular Immunology*. New York: Springer-Verlag, 1983–. Semi-monthly. ISSN 0724-6803.

204   *Journal of Neuroimmunology*. Amsterdam: Elsevier, 1981–. Bimonthly. ISSN 0165-5728.

205   *Journal of Reproductive Immunology*. Amsterdam: Elsevier, 1980–. Bimonthly. ISSN 0165-0371.

206   *Lancet*. London: The Lancet Ltd, 1823–. Weekly. ISSN 0023-7507.

207   *Ligand Review*. Houston: Technical and Professional Services, 1979–. Quarterly. ISSN 0197-4041.

208   *Lymphokine Research*. New York: Mary Ann Liebert, 1982–. Quarterly. ISSN 0277-6766.

209   *Medical Microbiology and Immunology*. New York: Springer-Verlag, 1886–. Quarterly. ISSN 0300-8584.

210   *Microbiology and Immunology* (formerly *Japanese Journal of Microbiology*). Tokyo: Japanese Society for Bacteriology, Japanese Society for Immunology, Japanese Society of Virology, 1957–. Bimonthly. ISSN 0021-5139.

211   *Molecular and Cellular Biochemistry*. The Hague: Dr W. Junk, 1981–. Bimonthly. ISSN 0300-8177.

212   *Molecular and Cellular Biology*. Philadelphia: American Society for Microbiology, 1981–. Monthly. ISSN 0270-7306.

213   *Molecular Immunology* (formerly *Immunochemistry*). New York: Pergamon Press, 1964–. Monthly. ISSN 0161-5890.

      Monoclonal Antibody Information, see Journal of Immunological Methods

214   *Monoclonal Antibody News*. New York: Mary Ann Liebert, 1981–. Bimonthly. ISSN 0272-4588.

215   *Natural Immunity and Cell Growth Regulation*. Basel: S. Karger, 1984–. Quarterly.

216   *Nature*. Basingstoke: Macmillan Journals Ltd, 1869–. Weekly. ISSN 0028-0836.

217   *Parasite Immunology*. Oxford: Blackwell Scientific Publications, 1979–. Bimonthly. ISSN 0141-9838.

218 *Proceedings of the National Academy of Sciences of the United States of America.* Washington, D.C.: National Academy of Sciences of the USA, 1915–. Semi-monthly. ISSN 0027-8424.

RES— The Journal of the Reticulo-endothelial Society, see Journal of Leukocyte Biology

219 *Scandinavian Journal of Immunology.* Oxford: Blackwell Scientific Publications, for the Scandinavian Society for Immunology, 1972–. Monthly. ISSN 0300-9475.

220 *Science.* Washington, D.C.: American Association for the Advancement of Science, 1848–. Weekly. ISSN 0036-8075.

221 *Soviet Immunology* (c/c *Immunologiya*). New York: Allerton Press, 1982–. Bimonthly. ISSN 0739-8433.

222 *Springer Seminars in Immunopathology.* New York: Springer-Verlag, 1978–. Quarterly. ISSN 0344-4325.

223 *Survey of Immunologic Research.* Basel: S. Karger, 1982–. Quarterly. ISSN 0252-9564.

224 *Thymus.* Amsterdam: Elsevier, 1979–. Bimonthly. ISSN 0165-6090.

225 *Tissue Antigens.* Copenhagen: Munksgaard, 1971–. 10 per yr. ISSN 0001-2815.

226 *Transplantation.* Baltimore: Williams & Wilkins, for the Transplantation Society, 1963–. Monthly. ISSN 0041-1337.

227 *Transplantation Proceedings.* New York: Grune & Stratton, for the Transplantation Society, 1969–. Quarterly. ISSN 0041-1345.

228 *Vaccine.* London: Butterworth Scientific Ltd, 1983–. Quarterly. ISSN 0264-410X.

229 *Veterinary Immunology and Immunopathology.* Amsterdam: Elsevier, 1980–. 6 per year. ISSN 0165-2427.

230 *Vox Sanguinis.* Basel: S. Karger, for the International Society for Blood Transfusion, 1951–. Monthly. ISSN 0042-9007.

Reviews *(see section 5.2)*

231 *Advances in Cancer Research.* New York: Academic Press, 1961–. Irregular. ISSN 0065-2776.

232 *Advances in Experimental Medicine and Biology.* New York: Plenum Press, 1967–. Irregular. ISSN 0065-2598.

233 *Advances in Immunology.* New York: Academic Press, 1961–. Irregular. ISSN 0065-2776.

234 *Advances in Inflammation Research.* New York: Raven Press, 1979–. Irregular.

235 *Advances in Veterinary Immunology.* Amsterdam: Elsevier, 1982–. Annual.

236 *American Lectures in Allergy and Immunology.* Springfield, Illinois: Charles C. Thomas, 1953. Irregular.

237 *Annual Review of Allergy*. New York: Medical Examination Publishing Co., 1973–. Annual. ISSN 0090-1083.

238 *Annual Review of Immunology*. Palo Alto, California: Annual Review Inc., 1983–. Biennial.

239 *Clinical Immunobiology*. New York: Academic Press, 1972–. Irregular.

240 *Contemporary Topics in Immunobiology*. New York: Plenum Press, 1972–. Irregular. ISSN 0093-4054.

241 *Contemporary Topics in Molecular Immunology*. New York: Plenum Press, 1972–. Irregular. ISSN 0090-8800.

242 *Contributions to Microbiology and Immunology*. Basel: S. Karger, 1973–. Irregular. ISSN 0301-3081.

243 *Current Topics in Immunology*. London: Edward Arnold, 1975–. Irregular. ISSN 0141-3368.

244 *Current Topics in Microbiology and Immunology*. New York: Springer Verlag, 1960–. Irregular (3–4 per year). ISSN 0070-2174.

245 *Developments in Biological Standardization*. Basel: S. Karger, 1955–. Irregular. ISSN 0301-5149.

246 *Developments in Immunology*. Amsterdam: Elsevier, 1978–. Irregular.

247 *Essays in Fundamental Immunology*. Oxford: Blackwell Scientific, 1973–1982. Irregular. ISSN 0301-4703.

248 *Human Cancer Immunology*. Amsterdam: Elsevier, 1980–. Irregular.

249 *Immunological Reviews*. Copenhagen: Munksgaard, 1969. Irregular (approx. 4 issues per year). ISSN 0105-2896.

250 *Immunology Reports and Reviews*. Darmstadt: DS Verlag, 1959–. Irregular. ISSN 0071-7908.

251 *Immunopathology*. New York: Grune & Stratton, 1959–. Irregular. ISSN 0073-5531. (Represents International Symposium on Immunopathology).

252 *Lymphokine Reports*. New York: Academic Press, 1980–. Annual. ISSN 0197-596X.

253 *Menarini Series on Immunopathology*. New York: Springer-Verlag, 1979–. Irregular.

254 *Methods in Enzymology*. New York: Academic Press, 1955–. Irregular. ISSN 0076-6879.

255 *Methods in Immunology and Immunochemistry*. New York: Academic Press. 1967. Irregular. ISSN 0076-6917.

256 *Perspectives in Immunology*. New York: Academic Press, 1969–. Irregular.

257 *Practical Methods in Clinical Immunology*. Edinburgh: Churchill Livingstone, 1980–. Irregular (3–4 per year).

258 *Progress in Allergy*. Basel: S. Karger, 1939–. Irregular. ISSN 0079–6034.

259 *Progress in Cancer Research and Therapy.* New York: Raven Press, 1976–. Irregular.

260 *Recent Advances in Clinical Immunology.* Edinburgh: Churchill Livingstone. 1983–. Irregular. ISSN 0140-6957.

261 *Techniques in Immunocytochemistry.* New York: Academic Press, 1982–. Irregular.

Monograph Serials

262 *The Antigens.* New York: Academic Press, 1973–. Irregular.

263 *Clinics in Immunology and Allergy.* Eastbourne: W. B. Saunders, 1981–. Three issues per year. ISSN 0260-4639.

264 *Comprehensive Immunology.* New York: Plenum Press, 1977–. Semi-annual. ISSN 0149-1148.

265 *Immunology: an International Series of Monographs and Treatises.* New York: Academic Press, 1967–. Irregular (every 2–3 years). ISSN 0076-6917.

266 *Immunology Series.* New York: Marcel Dekker, 1973–. Irregular (3–4 per year).

267 *Interferons.* New York: Academic Press, 1979–. Irregular.

267a *Lymphokines.* New York: Academic Press, 1980–. 213 per year.

268 *Monographs in Allergy.* Basel: S. Karger, 1966–. 2 per year. ISSN 0077-0760.

269 *Research Monographs in Immunology.* Amsterdam: Elsevier, 1980–. Irregular.

Books

Bibliographies Covering Books *(see* section 5.3)

270 *Book Review Index.* Detroit: Gale, 1965–. Bimonthly. ISSN 0524-0581.

271 *Books in Print.* New York: Bowker, 1948–. Annual. (Microfiche edition monthly or quarterly.) ISSN 0068-0214. On-line on BRS and DIALOG.

272 *British Books in Print.* London: Whitaker, 1874–. Annual (fiche edition monthly). ISSN 0068-1350. On-line on BLAISE-Line.

273 *British National Bibliography.* London: British Library, 1950–. Weekly. ISSN 0007-1544. On-line on BLAISE-Line.

274 Cassell *and* The Publishers Association. *Directory of publishing.* 10th edn. London: Cassell, 1983. ISBN 0-304-30913-3.

275 *Catline.* Bethesda, Maryland: National Library of Medicine, 1806–. Weekly updates. On-line on BLAISE-Link, National Library of Medicine and Dimdi.

276 *Index to Book Reviews in the Sciences.* Philadelphia: Institute for Scientific Information, 1980–. Quarterly.

277 *International ISBN publishers directory.* New York: Bowker, 1983. ISBN 3-88053-015-7.

278 *LC Marc.* Washington, D.C.: Library of Congress, 1968–. *Hosts:* DIALOG, BLAISE-Line.

279 *Marcfiche.* Washington, D.C.: Library of Congress, 1966–. Weekly.

280 *Medical Books and Serials in Print.* New York: Bowker, 1978–. Annual. ISSN 0000-0574.

281 National Library of Medicine. *Current Catalog.* Bethesda, Maryland: NLM, 1966–. Quarterly. ISSN 0090-3132.

282 *National Union Catalog (NUC) Books.* Washington, D.C.: Library of Congress, 1983–. Monthly updates (microfiche only). ISSN 0734-7650.

283 OCLC. Dublin, Ohio: OCLC, continual update.

284 *REMARC.* Arlington, Virginia: Carrollton Press, 1897–1978. Monthly updates. *Host:* DIALOG.

285 *RLIN.* Stanford, California: Research Libraries Group, continuous updates.

286 *Scientific and Technical Books and Serials in Print.* New York: Bowker, 1978–. Annual. ISSN 0000-054X.

287 *Subject Guide to Books in Print.* New York: Bowker, 1957–. Annual. ISSN 0000-0519.

288 *Subject Guide to Forthcoming Books.* New York: Bowker, 1957–. Monthly.

289 *UK Marc.* London: British Library, Bibliographic Services Division, 1950–. *Host:* BLAISE-Line.

290 *Whitaker's Classified Monthly Book List.* London: Whitaker, 1983–. Monthly. ISSN 0263-9432.

291 Wiley Catalogue. New York: John Wiley, 1940–. Bimonthly update. *Host:* DIALOG.

General

292 **Bach, J. F.** (Ed.). *Immunology.* 2nd edn. New York: John Wiley, 1982. (1032 pp.) ISBN 0-471-08044-6.

293 **Barret, J. T.** *Textbook of immunology: an introduction to immunochemistry and immunobiology.* 4th edn. St Louis: C. V. Mosby Co., 1983. (537 pp.) ISBN 0-801-60504-0.

294 **Baumgarten, A.** (Ed.). *Immunology.* (2 parts) Boca Raton, Florida: CRC Press, 1978, 1979. Part 1 (464 pp.), ISBN 0-8493-7021-3. Part 2 (480 pp.), ISBN 0-8493-7022-1.

295 **Benacerraf, B.** and **Unanue, E. F.** *Textbook of immunology.* (2nd edn. in preparation). Baltimore: Williams & Wilkins, 1979. (292 pp.) ISBN 0-683-00527-8.

296 **Bier, O. G., da Silva, W. D.** and **Goetze, D.** *Fundamentals of immunology.* New York: Springer-Verlag, 1981. (442 pp.) ISBN 0-387-90529-4.

297 **Bigley, N. J.** *Immunologic fundamentals*. 2nd edn. Chichester: Yearbook Medical Publishers, 1981. (341 pp.) ISBN 0-8151-0801-X.

298 **Clark, W. R.** *Experimental foundations of modern immunology*. Chichester: John Wiley, 1980 (372 pp.) ISBN 0-471-04088-6.

299 **Cooper, E. L.** *General immunology*. Oxford: Pergamon Press, 1982. (343 pp.) ISBN 0-08-026369-0.

300 **Doria, G.** and **Eshkol, A.** (Eds). *The immune system: functions and therapy of dysfunction*. New York: Academic Press, 1980. (293 pp.) ISBN 0-12-220550-2.

301 **Feinberg, G.** and **Jackson, M. A.** *The chain of immunology*. Oxford: Blackwell Scientific Publications, 1983. (86 pp.) ISBN 0-632-00881-4.

302 **Golub, E. S.** (Ed.). *Immunology: benchmark papers in microbiology*. (2 vols). London: Hutchinson Ross, 1981. Part 1 (372 pp.), ISBN 0-12-786546-2. Part 2 (270 pp.), ISBN 0-12-786547-0.

303 **Inchley, C. J.** *Immunobiology*. London: Edward Arnold, 1981. (88 pp.) ISBN 0-7131-2808-9.

304 **Klein, J.** *Immunology: the science of self–non-self discrimination*. Chichester: John Wiley, 1982. (687 pp.) ISBN 0-471-05124-1.

305 **Kwapinski, G.** and **Kwapinski, E. H.** (Eds). *The antigenicity of man*. Springfield, Illinois: Charles C. Thomas, 1981. (196 pp.) ISBN 0-398-04163-6.

306 **McConnell, I., Munro, A.** and **Waldmann, H.** *The immune system — a course on the molecular and cellular basis of immunity*. 2nd edn. Oxford: Blackwell Scientific Publications, 1981. (336 pp.) ISBN 0-632-00626-9.

306a **Myrvik, Q. N.** and **Welser, R. S.** (Eds). *Fundamentals of immunology*. 2nd edn. Philadelphia: Lea & Febiger, 1984. (510 pp.) ISBN 0-8121-0866-3.

307 **Nisonoff, A.** *Introduction to molecular immunology*. Oxford: Blackwell Scientific Publications, 1982. (224 pp.) ISBN 0-878-93594-0.

308 **Paul, W. E.** (Ed.). *Fundamental immunology*. New York: Raven Press, 1983. (880 pp.) ISBN 0-89004-923-8.

309 **Playfair, J. H. L.** *Immunology at a glance*. 2nd edn. Oxford: Blackwell Scientific Publications, 1982. (38 pp.) ISBN 0-632-00805-9.

310 **Roitt, I. M.** *Essential immunology*. 5th edn. Oxford: Blackwell Scientific Publications, 1984. (400 pp.) ISBN 0-632-01239-0.

311 **Rose, N. R., Milgrom, F.** and **Van Oss, C. J.** (Eds). *Principles of immunology*. 2nd edn. New York: Macmillan, 1979. (544 pp.) ISBN 0-02-403610-2.

312 **Steinberg, C. M.** and **Lefkovits, I.** (Eds). *The immune system:* vol. 1, *Past and future*; vol. 2, *The present*. Basel: S. Karger, 1981. (Vol. 1, 460 pp., Vol. 2, 492 pp.), ISBN 3-8055-3409-4.

313 **Stites, D. P., Stobo, J. D., Fudenberg, H. H.** and **Wells, J. V.** (Eds). *Basic and clinical immunology.* 4th edn. Los Altos, California: Lange Medical Publications, 1982. (778 pp.) ISBN 0-87041-223-X.

313a **Weir, D. M.** *Immunology: an outline for students of medicine and biology.* Edinburgh: Churchill Livingstone, 1983. (255 pp.) ISBN 0-443-02840-0.

History

314 **Humphrey, J. H.** and **White, R. G.** *Immunology for students of medicine.* 3rd edn, pp. 1–34. Oxford: Blackwell Scientific Publications, 1970. ISBN 0-632-02180-7.

315 **Silverstein, A. M.** History of immunology: development of the concept of immunologic specificity. Part I, *Cellular Immunology* **67,** 396 (1982); Part II, *Cellular Immunology* **71,** 183 (1982); Part III, *Cellular Immunology* **78,** 174 (1983); Part IV, *Cellular Immunology* **80,** 416 (1983).

316 **Wilson, D.** *The science of self,* pp. 95–129. London: Longman, 1972. ISBN 0-582-12776-9.

317 *See* Books, General, for works by **Cooper, E. L.** (1982); **Golub, E. S.** (1981); **Klein, J.** (1982); and **Steinberg, C. M.** and **Lefkovits, I.** (1981).

Allergy, Autoimmunity and Hypersensitivity

318 **Asthma and Allergy Foundation of America** and **Norback, C. T.** (Eds). *The allergy encyclopaedia.* Chichester: Year Book Medical Publishers, 1981. (267 pp.) ISBN 0-452-25345-4.

319 **Dukor, P., Kallos, P., Schlumberger, H. D.** and **West, G. B.** (Eds). *Pseudo-allergic reactions: involvement of drugs and chemicals.* Vol. 1, *Genetic aspects and anaphylactoid reactions.* Basel: S. Karger, 1980. (324 pp.) ISBN 3-8055-0537-X.

320 **Goetzl, E. J.** and **Kay, A. B.** (Eds). *Contemporary issues in clinical immunology and allergy.* Vol. 1, *Current perspective in allergy.* London: Churchill Livingstone, 1982. (195 pp.) ISBN 0-443-02503-7.

321 **Lessof, M. H.** (Ed.). *Immunological and clinical aspects of allergy.* Lancaster: MTP Press, 1981. (452 pp.) ISBN 0-85200-244-0.

322 **Maini, R. N.** and **Berry, H.** (Eds). *Modulation of autoimmunity and disease: the penicillamine experience.* New York: Praeger Scientific, 1981. (324 pp.) ISBN 0-03-659627-0.

323 **Middleton, E., Ellis, E. F.** and **Reed, C. E.** (Eds). *Allergy: principles and practice.* 2nd edn. Oxford: Blackwell Scientific Publications, 1984. (423 pp.) ISBN 0-8016-3419-9.

324 **Mygind, N.** *Nasal allergy.* (2nd edn.) Oxford: Blackwell Scientific Publications, 1984. (350 pp.) ISBN 0-632-01188-2.

325 **Pinchera, A., Fenzi, G. F.** and **Baschieri, L.** (Eds). *Autoimmune aspects of endocrine disorders.* New York: Academic Press, 1981. (434 pp.). ISBN 0-12-556750-2.

326 **Piper, P. J.** (Ed.). *SRS — A and leukotrines*. Chichester: John Wiley, 1981. (290 pp.). ISBN 0471-27959-5.

327 **Talal, N.** (Ed.). *Autoimmunity*. New York: Academic Press, 1977. (734 pp.) ISBN 0-12-682350-2.

328 **Volpé, R.** *Autoimmunity in the endocrine system*. New York: Springer-Verlag, 1981. (197 pp.) ISBN 0-387-10677-4.

Cellular Immunology and Cytotoxicity

329 **Aiuti, F.** and **Wigzell, H.** (Eds). *Thymus, thymic hormones and T-lymphocytes*. New York: Academic Press, 1980. (445 pp.) ISBN 0-12-046450-0.

330 **Bach, F. H., Bonavida, B., Vitetta, E.** and **Fox, C. F.** (Eds). *T- and B-lymphocytes: recognition and function*. New York: Academic Press, 1979. (709 pp.) ISBN 0-12-069850-1.

331 **Cohen, S.** and **Oppenheim, J.** (Eds). *Biology of the lymphokines*. New York: Academic Press, 1979. (656 pp.) ISBN 0-12-178250-6.

332 **Constantin, A. B.** (Ed.). *Idiotypes and lymphocytes*. New York: Academic Press, 1981. (211 pp.) ISBN 0-12-112950-0.

333 **Fauci, A. S.** and **Ballieux, R. E.** *Human B-lymphocyte function*. London: Raven Press, 1982. ISBN 0-89004-620-4.

334 **Forster, O.** and **Landy, M.** (Eds.). *Heterogeneity of mononuclear phagocytes*. New York: Academic Press, 1981. (538 pp.) ISBN 0-12-262360-6.

335 **Gadebusch, H. H.** (Ed.). *Phagocytes and cellular immunity*. Boca Raton, Florida: CRC Press, 1979. (176 pp.) ISBN 0-8493-5349-1.

336 **Golub, E. S.** *The cellular basis of the immune response*. Oxford: Blackwell Scientific Publications, 1981. (340 pp.) ISBN 0-87893-212-7.

337 **Goodwin, J. S.** (Ed.). *Suppressor cells in human disease*. New York: Marcel Dekker, 1981. (363 pp.) ISBN 0-8247-1290-0.

338 **Hadden, J. W.** and **Stowart, W. E.** (Eds). *The lymphokines — biochemistry and biological activity*. Clifton, New Jersey: Humana Press, 1981. (452 pp.) ISBN 0-896-03012-1.

339 **Herberman, R. B.** (Ed.). *NK cells and other natural effector cells*. New York: Academic Press, 1982. (1608 pp.) ISBN 0-12-341360-5.

340 **Inglis, J. R.** (Ed.). *T-lymphocytes today*. Cambridge: Elsevier Biomedical, 1983. (200 pp.) ISBN 0-444-80524-9.

341 **Inglis, J. R.** (Ed.). *B-lymphocytes today*. Cambridge: Elsevier Biomedical, 1982. (165 pp.) ISBN 0-444-80454-4.

342 **Luderer, A. A.** and **Weetall, H. H.** (Eds). *Clinical cellular immunology — molecular and therapeutic reviews*. Clifton, New Jersey: Human Press, 1982. (389 pp.) ISBN 0-876-03011-3.

343 **Oppenheim, J. J.** and **Cohen, S.** (Eds). *Interleukins, lymphokines and cytokines*. New York: Academic Press, 1983. (824 pp.) ISBN 0-12-527540-4.

344 **Pernis, B.** and **Vogel, J. H.** (Eds). *Regulatory T-lymphocytes.* New York: Academic Press, 1980. (449 pp.) ISBN 0-12-551860-9.

345 **Sato, V. L.** and **Gefter, M. L.** (Eds). *Cellular immunology (selected readings and critical commentary).* Reading, Massachusetts: Addison Wesley, 1981.

346 **de Sousa, M.** *Lymphocyte circulation, experimental and clinical aspects.* Chichester: Wiley Interscience, 1981. (259 pp.) ISBN 0-471-27854-8.

347 **Unanue, E. R.** and **Rosenthal, A. S.** (Eds). *Macrophage regulation of immunity.* New York: Academic Press, 1980. (523 pp.) ISBN 0-12-708550-5.

Clinical Immunology

348 **Bach, F. H.** and **Good, R. A.** (Eds). *Clinical immunobiology,* 4 vols. New York: Academic Press. Vol. 1, 1972 (296 pp.) ISBN 0-12-070001-8. Vol. 2, 1974 (312 pp.) ISBN 0-12-070002-6. Vol. 3, 1976 (442 pp.) ISBN 0-12-070003-4. Vol. 4, 1980 (198 pp.) ISBN 0-12-070004-2.

349 **Basten, A.** (Ed.) *Clinical immunology in medical practice.* Oxford: Blackwell Scientific Publications, 1981. (360 pp.) ISBN 0-632-00203-4.

349a **Chapel, H. M.** and **Haeney, M. R.** *Essentials of clinical immunology.* Oxford: Blackwell Scientific Publications, 1984. In preparation.

350 **Clancy, R.** and **Bienenstock, J.** *Concepts in clinical immunology.* Oxford: Blackwell Scientific Publications, 1983. (240 pp.) ISBN 0-86793-072-1.

351 **Fikrig, S. M.** (Ed.) *Handbook of immunology for students and house staff.* Weinheim: Verlag Chemie, 1982. (216 pp.) ISBN 0-89573-111-8.

352 **Franklin, E. C.** (Ed.). *Clinical immunology update: review for physicians.* Cambridge: Elsevier Biomedical, 1983. (409 pp.) ISBN 0-444-00711-3.

353 **Holborow, E. J.** and **Reeves, W. G.** (Eds). *Immunology in medicine: a comprehensive guide to clinical immunology.* 2nd edn. New York: Academic Press, 1983. (676 pp.) ISBN 0-8089-1573-8.

354 **Lachmann, P. J.** and **Peters, D. K.** (Eds). *Clinical aspects of immunology.* 4th edn. 2 vols. Oxford: Blackwell Scientific Publications, 1982. (Vol. 1, 794 pp. Vol. 2, 1041 pp.), ISBN 0-632-00702-8.

355 **Reeves, W. G.** *Lecture notes on clinical immunology.* Oxford: Blackwell Scientific Publications, 1981. (304 pp.) ISBN 0-632-00776-1.

356 **Richter, M.** *Clinical immunology: a physician's guide.* 2nd edn. Baltimore: Williams & Wilkins, 1981. (328 pp.) ISBN 0-683-07255-2.

357 **Turk, J. L.** and **Collins, W.** *Immunology in clinical medicine.* London: Heinemann, 1978. (265 pp.) ISBN 0-433-32852-5.

Developmental Immunology

358 **Cooper, E. L.** and **Brazier, M. A. B.** (Eds). *Developmental immunology: clinical problems and aging.* New York: Academic Press, 1982. (321 pp.) ISBN 0-12-188040-0.

359 **Fabris, N.** (Ed.). *Immunology and aging.* Amsterdam: Martinus Nijhoff, 1982. (240 pp.) ISBN 90-247-2640-9.

360 **Kay, K. M. B.** and **Makinodan, T.** *CRC Handbook of immunology in aging.* Boca Raton, Florida: CRC Press, 1981. (328 pp.) ISBN 0-8493-3144-7.

Immune Response and Immunoglobulins

361 **Delisi, C.** and **Hiernaux, J. R.** *Regulation of immune response dynamics.* 2 vols. Boca Raton, Florida: CRC Press, 1982. Vol. 1 (176 pp.) ISBN 0-8493-6632-1. Vol. 2 (184 pp.) ISBN 0-8493-6633-X.

361a **Froese, A.** and **Paraskevas, F.** *Structure and function of Fc receptors.* New York: Marcel Dekker, 1983. 294 pp. ISBN 0-8247-1814-3.

362 **Janeway, C., Sercarz, E. E.** and **Wigzell, H.** *Immunoglobulin idiotypes.* New York: Academic Press, 1981. (902 pp.) ISBN 0-12-380380-2.

363 **Sercarz, E.** and **Cunningham, A. J.** (Eds). *Strategies of immune regulation.* New York: Academic Press, 1980. (537 pp.) ISBN 0-12-637140-7.

363a **Steward, M. W.** *Antibodies: their structure and function.* London: Chapman & Hall, 1984. (96 pp.) ISBN 0-412-25640-1.

364 **Strober, W., Hanson, L. A.** and **Sell, K. W.** (Eds). *Recent advances in mucosal immunity.* New York: Raven Press, 1982. (453 pp.) ISBN 0-890-04642-5.

Immunity to Infection

365 **Barriga, O. O.** *The immunology of parasitic infections.* Lancaster: MTP Press, 1981. (276 pp.) ISBN 0-8391-1621-7.

365a **Ennis, F. A.** (Ed.). *Human immunity to viruses.* New York: Academic Press, 1983. (363 pp.) ISBN 0-12-239980-3.

366 **Koprowski, C.** and **Koprowski, H.** (Eds). *Viruses and immunity.* New York: Academic Press, 1975. (156 pp.) ISBN 0-12-420350-7.

367 **Lambert, H. P.** and **Wood, C. B. S.** (Eds). *Immunological aspects of infection in the fetus and newborn.* New York: Academic Press, 1981. (249 pp.) ISBN 0-12-434660-X.

368 **Larralde, C.** (Ed.). *Molecules, cells and parasites in immunology.* New York: Academic Press, 1980. (231 pp.) ISBN 0-12-436840-9.

369 **McLean, D. M.** *Immunological investigation of human virus diseases.* London: Churchill Livingstone, 1983. (112 pp.) ISBN 0-443-02536-3.

370 **Mansfield, J. M.** (Ed.). *Parasitic diseases.* Vol. 1, *The immunology.* New York: Marcel Dekker, 1981. (323 pp.) ISBN 0-8247-1409-1.

371 **Mims, C. A.** and **White, D. O.** *Viral pathogenesis and immunology.* Oxford: Blackwell Scientific Publications, 1984. (300 pp.) ISBN 0-632-01193-9.

372 **Notkins, A. C.** (Ed.) *Viral immunology and immunopathology.* New York: Academic Press, 1975. (498 pp.) ISBN 0-12-522050-2.

373   **Strickland, G. T.** and **Hunter, K. W.** (Eds). *Immunoparasitology: principles and methods in malaria and schistosomiasis research.* New York: Praeger, 1982. (336 pp.) ISBN 0-030-61499-6.

374   **Woolcock, J. B.** *Bacterial infection and immunity.* Amsterdam: Elsevier, 1979. (220 pp.) ISBN 0-444-41768-0.

Immunogenetics, HLA and MHC

375   **Braun, W. E.** *HLA and disease.* Boca Raton, Florida: CRC Press, 1979. (160 pp.) ISBN 0-8493-5795-0.

376   **Dorf, M. E.** (Ed.). *The role of the major histocompatibility complex in immunobiology.* Chichester: John Wiley, 1982. (416 pp.) ISBN 0-471-10124-9.

377   **Hildemann, W. H.** *Comprehensive immunogenetics.* Oxford: Blackwell Scientific Publications, 1981. (384 pp.) ISBN 0-632-00788-5.

378   **Hildemann, W. H.** (Ed.). *Frontiers in immunogenetics.* New York: Elsevier, 1981. (280 pp.) ISBN 0-444-00624-9.

379   **Miller, W. V.** and **Rodey, G.** *HLA without tears.* New York: Raven Press, 1981. (167 pp.) ISBN 0-89189-084-X.

379a **Möller, E.** and **Möller, G.** *Genetics of the immune response.* New York: Plenum Press, 1983. (324 pp.) ISBN 0-306-41252-7.

380   **Williamson, A. R.** and **Turner, M. W.** *Essential immunogenetics.* Oxford: Blackwell Scientific Publications, 1981. (240 pp.) ISBN 0-632-00236-0.

380a **Zaleski, M. B., Dubiski, S., Niles, E. G.** and **Cunningham, R. K.** *Immunogenetics.* Marshfield, Massachusetts: Pitman, 1983. (514 pp.) ISBN 0-273-01925-2.

Immunohaematology

381   **Bryant, N. J.** *An introduction to immunohaematology.* 2nd edn. Eastbourne: W. B. Saunders, 1982. (350 pp.) ISBN 0-7216-2167-8.

382   **Nyedegger, V. E.** (Ed.). *Immunotherapy: a guide to immunoglobulin prophylaxis and therapy.* New York: Academic Press, 1982. (490 pp.) ISBN 0-12-523280-2.

Immunopathology

383   **Altura, B. M.** and **Salba, T. M.** (Eds). *Pathophysiology of the reticuloendothelial system.* New York: Raven Press, 1981. (248 pp.) ISBN 0-89004-441-4.

384   **Amos, D. B., Schwartz, R. S.** and **Janicki, B. W.** (Eds). *Immune mechanisms and disease.* New York: Academic Press, 1979. (376 pp.) ISBN 0-12-055850-5.

385   **Asherson, G. L.** and **Webster, A. D. B.** *Diagnosis and treatment of immuno-deficiency disease.* Oxford: Blackwell Scientific Publications, 1980. (400 pp.) ISBN 0-632-00183-6.

386 **Cummings, N. B.** and **Michael, A. F.** (Eds). *Immune mechanisms in renal disease.* New York: Plenum Medical Book Co., 1983. (564 pp.) ISBN 0-306-40948-8.

387 **Dixon, F. J.** and **Fisher, D. W.** (Eds). *Immunopathology.* Oxford: Blackwell Scientific Publications. In preparation.

388 **Dixon, F. J.** and **Fisher, D. W.** (Eds). *The biology of immunologic disease.* Oxford: Blackwell Scientific Publications, 1983. (384 pp.) ISBN 0-87893-148-1.

389 **Farid, N. R.** *HLA in endocrine and metabolic disorder.* New York: Academic Press, 1981. (357 pp.) ISBN 0-12-247780-4.

390 **Glynn, L. E.** and **Reading, C. A.** *Immunological investigation of connective tissue disease.* London: Churchill Livingstone, 1981. (108 pp.) ISBN 0-443-01850-2.

391 **Goos, M.** and **Christophers, E.** (Eds). *Lymphoproliferative diseases of the skin.* New York: Springer-Verlag, 1982. (311 pp.) ISBN 3-540-11222-7.

392 **Hokama, Y.** and **Nakamura, R. M.** *Immunology and immunopathology: basic concepts.* Boston, Massachusetts: Little, Brown, 1982. (528 pp.) ISBN 0-316-36932-2.

393 **Irvine, J.** (Ed.). *Immunology of diabetes.* Edinburgh: Teviot Scientific Publications Limited, 1981. (377 pp.) ISBN 0-906341-01-9.

394 **Klopper, A.** (Ed.). *Immunology of the human placenta.* New York: Praeger, 1982. (136 pp.) ISBN 0-03-062117-8.

394a **Lessof, M. M.** (Ed.). *Immunology of cardiovascular disease.* New York: Marcel Dekker, 1981. (448 pp.) ISBN 0-8247-1513-6.

395 **Roitt, I. M.** and **Lehner, T.** *Immunology of oral diseases.* Oxford: Blackwell Scientific Publications, 1980. (480 pp.) ISBN 0-632-00613-7.

396 **Sharma, R. P.** and **Street, J. C.** (Eds). *Immunologic considerations in toxicology.* Boca Raton, Florida: CRC Press, 1980. (256 pp.) ISBN 0-8493-5271-1.

397 **Thomas, H. C.** and **Jewell, D. P.** *Clinical gastrointestinal immunology.* Oxford: Blackwell Scientific Publications, 1979. (276 pp.) ISBN 0-632-00022-8.

398 **Thomas, H. C., Miescher, P. A.** and **Mueller-Eberhard, H. J.** (Eds). *Immunological aspects of liver disease.* New York: Springer Verlag, 1982. (208 pp.) ISBN 0-387-11310-X.

399 **Ward, P. A.** (Ed.). *Immunology of inflammation.* Amsterdam: Elsevier Science Publishers, 1983. (422 pp.) ISBN 0-444-8000-0.

400 **Weigle, W. O.** (Ed.). *Advances in immunopathology.* London: Edward Arnold, 1981. (500 pp. approx.) ISBN 0-7131-4395-9.

401 **Zabriskie, J. B., Fillit, H., Villareal, H.** and **Becker, E. L.** (Eds). *Clinical immunology of the kidney.* New York: John Wiley, 1982. (453 pp.) ISBN 0-471-02675-1.

Interferon

401a **Burke, D. C.** and **Morris, A. G.** *Interferons.* Cambridge: Cambridge University Press, 1983. (337 pp.) ISBN 0-521-25069-2.

402 **Friedman, R. M.** *Interferon: a primer.* New York: Academic Press, 1981. (151 pp.) ISBN 0-12-268280-7.

403 **Gresser, I.** (Ed.). *Interferon.* New York: Academic Press. Vol. 1, 1979 (163 pp.) ISBN 0-12-302250-9. Vol. 2, 1981 (112 pp.) ISBN 0-12-302251-7. Vol. 3, 1982 (164 pp.) ISBN 0-12-302252-5. Vol. 4, 1983 (150 pp.) ISBN 0-12-302253-3. Vol. 5, 1984 (248 pp.) ISBN 0-12-302254-1.

404 **Merigan, T. C.** and **Friedman, R. M.** (Eds). *Interferons.* New York: Academic Press, 1982. (512 pp.) ISBN 0-12-491220-6.

405 **Sikora, K.** (Ed.). *Interferon and cancer.* New York: Plenum Press, 1983. (223 pp.) ISBN 0-306-41379-5.

Monoclonal Antibodies (Hybridoma Technology)

406 **Albertini, A.** and **Ekins, R.** (Eds). *Monoclonal antibodies and developments in immunoassay.* New York: Elsevier/North-Holland, 1981. (417 pp.) ISBN 0-444-80373-4.

406a **Boss, B. D., Langman, R., Trowbridge, I.** and **Dulbecco, R.** (Eds). *Monoclonal antibodies and cancer.* New York: Academic Press, 1984. (328 pp.) ISBN 0-12-118880-9.

407 **Garrison-Fathman, C.** and **Fitch, F. W.** (Eds). *Isolation, characterization and utilization of T-lymphocyte clones.* New York: Academic Press, 1982. (576 pp.) ISBN 0-12-243320-4.

407a **Goding, J. W.** *Monoclonal antibodies: principles and practice.* New York: Academic Press, 1983. (288 pp.) ISBN 0-12-287020-4.

407b **Greaves, M.** (Ed.). *Monoclonal antibodies to receptors.* London: Chapman & Hall, 1984. (250 pp.) ISBN 0-412-25330-5.

407c **Haynes, B. F.** and **Eisenbarth, G. S.** *Monoclonal antibodies: probes for the study of autoimmunity and immunodeficiency.* New York: Academic Press, 1984. (344 pp.) ISBN 0-12-334880-3.

408 **Houba, V.** and **Chan, S. H.** (Eds). *Properties of the monoclonal antibodies produced by hybridoma technology and their application to the study of diseases.* Geneva: UNDP/World Bank/WHO, 1982. (199 pp.).

409 **Hurrel, J. G. R.** (Ed.). *Monoclonal hybridoma antibodies: techniques and applications.* Boca Raton, Florida: CRC Press, 1982. (240 pp.) ISBN 0-8493-6511-2.

410 **Katz, D. H.** (Ed.). *Monoclonal antibodies and T-cell products.* Boca Raton, Florida: CRC Press, 1982. (184 pp.) ISBN 0-8493-6580-5.

411 **Kennett, R. H., McLean, T. J.** and **Bechtol, K. B.** (Eds). *Monoclonal antibodies. Hybridomas: a new dimension in biological analyses.* New York: Plenum Press, 1980. (423 pp.) ISBN 0-306-40408-7.

412 **Kohler, G.** and **EMBO** (Eds). *Hybridoma techniques* (EMBO/SKMB course 1980, Basel). New York: Cold Spring Harbor Laboratory, 1980. (84 pp.) ISBN 0-87969-143-3.

413 **Løvberg, U.** *Monoclonal antibodies: production and maintenance.* London: Heinemann Medical Books, 1982. (66 pp.) ISBN 0-433-19645-9.

414 **McKay, R., Raff, M. C.** and **Reichardt, L. F.** (Eds). *Monoclonal antibodies to neural antigens.* New York: Cold Spring Harbor Laboratory, 1981. (297 pp.) ISBN 0-87969-138-7.

415 **McMichael, A.** and **Fabre, J.** (Eds). *Monoclonal antibodies in clinical medicine.* New York: Academic Press, 1982. (672 pp.) ISBN 0-12-485580-6.

416 **Sato, V. L.** (Ed.). *Monoclonal antibodies: a technology for industry and medicine.* Menlo Park, California: Benjamin/Cummings Publishing Co. In preparation.

417 **Sikora, K.** and **Smedley, H.** *Monoclonal antibodies.* Oxford: Blackwell Scientific Publications, 1984. (120 pp.) ISBN 0-632-01166-1.

Neuroimmunology and Immunopharmacology

418 **Ader, R.** (Ed.). *Psychoneuroimmunology.* New York: Academic Press, 1981. (684 pp.) ISBN 0-12-043780-5.

419 **Behan, P. O.** and **Currie, S.** *Clinical neuroimmunology. Major problems in neurology,* Vol. 8. Philadelphia: W. B. Saunders, 1978. (213 pp.) ISBN 0-7216-1672-0.

420 **Behan, P. O., terMeulen, V.** and **Rose, C. F.** (Eds). *Immunology of nervous system infections.* Amsterdam: Elsevier Scientific Publishers, 1983. (409 pp.) ISBN 0-444-80443-9.

421 **Brockes, J.** (Ed.). *Neuroimmunology.* New York: Plenum Press, 1982. (256 pp.) ISBN 0-306-40955-0.

422 **Dale, M. M.** and **Foreman, J. C.** (Eds). *Textbook of immunopharmacology.* Oxford: Blackwell Scientific Publications, 1983. (350 pp.) ISBN 0-632-00859-8.

422a **Hadden, J. W., Chedid, L., Dukor, P., Spreafico, F.** and **Willoughby, D.** (Eds). *Advances in immunopharmacology 2.* New York: Pergamon, 1983. (878 pp.) ISBN 0-08-029775-7.

423 **Rose, C. F.** *Clinical neuroimmunology.* Oxford: Blackwell Scientific Publications, 1979. (544 pp.) ISBN 0-632-00482-7.

424 **Rola-Pleszczynski, M.** and **Sirois, P.** (Eds). *Immunopharmacology.* Amsterdam: Elsevier Biomedical, 1982. (426 pp.) ISBN 0-444-80461-1.

425 **Webb, D. R.** *Immunopharmacology and the regulation of leukocyte function.* New York: Marcel Dekker, 1982. (312 pp.) ISBN 0-8247-1707-4.

Techniques (Including Immunochemistry)

425a **Aloisi, R. M.** and **Huyn, J.** (Eds). *Immunodiagnostics.* New York: Alan R. Liss, 1983. (304 pp.) ISBN 0-8451-1657-6.

426 **Axelsen, N. H.** (Ed.). *Handbook of immunoprecipitation in gel techniques.* Oxford: Blackwell Scientific Publications, 1983. (394 pp.) ISBN 0-632-01057-6.

427 **Bernard, A., Boumsell, L., Dausset, J., Milstein, C.** and **Schlossman, S. F.** (Eds). *Leukocyte typing.* Berlin: Springer-Verlag, 1984. (820 pp.) ISBN 3-540012-56-4.

428 **Clausen, J.** *Immunological techniques for the identification and estimation of macromolecules.* 2nd edn. New York: Elsevier, 1981. (401 pp.) ISBN 0-444-80244-4.

429 **Cline, M. J.** (Ed.). *Leukocyte function.* New York: Churchill Livingstone, 1981. (150 pp.) ISBN 0-686-28872-6.

430 **Cuello, A. C.** (Ed.). *Immunohistochemistry.* New York: John Wiley, 1983. (500 pp.) ISBN 0-471-10245-8.

431 **Holborrow, E. J.** and **Johnson, G. D.** *Atlas of auto-antibody immunofluorescence: a guide to recognition of tissue staining patterns.* Oxford: Blackwell Scientific Publications, 1981. (240 pp.) ISBN 0-632-00343-X.

432 **Hudson, L.** and **Hay, F. C.** *Practical immunology.* Oxford: Blackwell Scientific Publications, 1980. 2nd edn. (359 pp.) ISBN 0-632-00353-7.

433 **Johnstone, A.** and **Thorpe, R.** *Immunochemistry in practice.* Oxford: Blackwell Scientific Publications, 1982. (312 pp.) ISBN 0-632-00836-9.

434 **Kwapinski, G.** *The methodology of investigative and clinical immunology.* Melbourne, Florida: Robert E. Krieger Publishing Co., 1982. (523 pp.) ISBN 0-882-75828-4.

435 **Leftovits, I.** and **Pernis, B.** (Eds). *Immunological methods.* 2 vols. New York: Academic Press. Vol. 1, 1979 (467 pp.) ISBN 0-12-442750-2. Vol. 2, 1981 (316 pp.) ISBN 0-12-442702-2.

436 **Maggio, E. T.** (Ed.). *Enzyme-immunoassay.* Boca Raton, Florida: CRC Press, 1980. (295 pp.) ISBN 0-8493-5617-2.

437 **Marchalonis, J. T.** and **Warr, G. W.** (Eds). *Antibody as a tool: the applications of immunochemistry.* Chichester: John Wiley, 1982. (578 pp.) ISBN 0-471-10084-6.

438 **Mishell, B. B.** and **Shiigi, S. M.** (Eds). *Selected methods in cellular immunology.* San Francisco: W. H. Freeman, 1980. (486 pp.) ISBN 0-7167-1106-0.

439 **Parrat, D., McKenzie, H., Nielsen, K. H.** and **Cobb, S. J.** *Radioimmunoassay of antibody and its clinical application.* Chichester: John Wiley, 1982. (174 pp.) ISBN 0-471-10061-7.

440 **Polak, J. M.** and **Van Noorden, S.** (Eds). *Immunocytochemistry: Practical applications in pathology and biology.* Littleton, Massachusetts: John Wright, 1983. (395 pp.) ISBN 0-471-10010-2.

441 **Rose, N. R.** and **Friedman, H.** (Eds). *Manual of clinical immunology.* 2nd edn. Washington, D.C.: ASM, 1980. (1105 pp.) ISBN 0-914826-27-1.

441a **Talwar, G. P.** (Ed.). *A handbook of practical immunology.* New Delhi: Vikas, 1983. (533 pp.) ISBN 0-7069-1888-6.

442 **Thompson, R. A.** (Ed.). *Techniques in clinical immunology.* Oxford: Blackwell Scientific Publications, 1981. (280 pp.) ISBN 0-632-00723-0.

443 **Thomson, D. M. P.** (Ed.). *Assessment of immune status by the leukocyte adherence inhibition test.* New York: Academic Press, 1982. (398 pp.) ISBN 0-12-689750-6.

444 **Weir, D. M.** (Ed.). *Handbook of experimental immunology.* 3rd edn. 3 vols. Oxford: Blackwell Scientific Publications, 1978. Vol. 1, *Immunochemistry* (534 pp.) ISBN 0-632-00166-6. Vol. 2, *Cellular immunology* (350 pp.) ISBN 0-632-00176-3. Vol. 3, *Application of immunological methods* (348 pp.) ISBN 0-632-00186-0.

445 **Wick, G., Traill, K. N.** and **Schauenstein, K.** (Eds). *Immunofluorescence technology (selected theoretical and clinical aspects).* Amsterdam: Elsevier Biomedical, 1983. (460 pp.) ISBN 0-444-80398-X.

Transplantation, Immunosuppression and Immunotolerance

446 **Battisto, J. R.** and **Clamon, H. N.** (Eds). *Immunological tolerance to self and non-self.* New York: New York Academy of Sciences, 1982. (436 pp.) ISBN 0-89766-174-5.

447 **Calne, R. Y.** (Ed.). *Liver transplantation.* New York: Academic Press, 1983. ISBN 0-12-790767-X.

448 **Calne, R. Y.** (Ed.). *Transplantation immunology.* Oxford: Oxford University Press, 1984. (600 pp.) ISBN 0-19-261414-2.

449 **Gale, R. P., Fox, C. F.** and **Stusser, F. J. (Eds).** *Biology of bone marrow transplantation.* New York: Academic Press, 1980. (566 pp.) ISBN 0-12-273960-4.

450 **Hamburger, J., Crosnier, J., Bach, J. F.** and **Kreis, H.** (Eds). *Renal transplantation: theory and practice.* Baltimore: Williams & Wilkins, 1981. (384 pp.) ISBN 0-686-3872-9.

451 **Hraba, T.** and **Hasek, M.** (Eds). *Cellular and molecular mechanisms of immunologic tolerance.* New York: Marcel Dekker, 1981. (570 pp.) ISBN 0-8247-1552-7.

452 **Okunewick, J. P.** and **Meredith, R. F.** (Eds). *Graft versus leukemia in man and animal models.* Boca Raton, Florida: CRC Press, 1981. (304 pp.) ISBN 0-8493-5745-4.

453 **Salaman, J. R.** *Immunosuppressive therapy (The Current Status of Modern Therapy* series). Lancaster: MTP Press, 1981. (257 pp.) ISBN 0-85200-338-2.

Tumour Immunology

454 **Blasecki, J. W.** (Ed.). *Mechanisms of immunity to virus-induced cancers.* New York: Marcel Dekker, 1981. (365 pp.) ISBN 0-8247-1162-9.

455 **Busch, H.** and **Yeoman, L. C.** (Eds). *Tumor markers* (Vol. 20 of *Methods in Cancer Research*). New York: Academic Press, 1982. (423 pp.) ISBN 0-12-147679-0.

456   **Catovsky, D.** (Ed.). *The leukemic cell.* London: Churchill Livingstone, 1981. (288 pp.) ISBN 0-443-01911-8.

457   **Chirigos, M. A., Mitchell, M., Mastrangelo, M. J.** and **Krim, M.** (Eds). *Mediation of cellular immunity in cancer by immune modifiers.* New York: Raven Press, 1981. (287 pp.) ISBN 0-89004-628-X.

458   **Haller, O.** (Ed.). *Natural resistance to tumors and viruses.* Berlin: Springer Verlag, 1981. (128 pp.) ISBN 3-540-10732-0.

459   **Herberman, R. B.** (Ed.). *Natural cell mediated immunity against tumors.* New York: Academic Press, 1980. (1321 pp.) ISBN 0-12-341350-8.

460   **Prasad, N.** (Ed.). *Radiotherapy and cancer immunology.* Boca Raton, Florida: CRC Press, 1981. (216 pp.) ISBN 0-8493-5901-5.

461   **Richards, V.** (Ed.). *Current cancer immunology.* Basel: S. Karger, 1980. (295 pp.) ISBN 0-8055-3033-1.

462   **Terry, W. D.** and **Rosenberg, S. A.** (Eds). *Immunotherapy of human cancer.* Amsterdam: Excerpta Medica, 1982. (517 pp.) ISBN 0-444-00614-1.

463   **Vitetta, E. S.** (Ed.). *B- and T-cell tumors: biological and clinical aspects.* New York: Academic Press, 1983. (616 pp.) ISBN 0-12-722380-0.

Vaccination and Vaccines

464   **Duffy, J. I.** (Ed.). *Vaccine preparation techniques.* Park Ridge, New Jersey: Noyes Data Corp., 1980. (403 pp.) ISBN 0-8155-0796-8.

465   **Fulginiti, V. A.** (Ed.). *Immunization in clinical practice. (A useful guideline to vaccines, sera and immune globulin in clinical practice.)* New York: Harper & Row, 1982. (302 pp.) ISBN 0-397-50539-6.

465a   **Germanier, P.** (Ed.). *Bacterial vaccines.* New York: Academic Press, 1984. (456 pp.) ISBN 0-12-28088-0.

466   **Mizrahi, A., Hertman, I., Klinberg, M. A.** and **Kohn, A.** (Eds). *New developments with human and veterinary vaccines.* London: Heyden, 1980. (444 pp.) ISBN 0-8451-0047-5.

Veterinary Immunology

467   **Hay, J. B.** (Ed.). *Animal models of immunological processes.* New York: Academic Press, 1982. ISBN 0-12-333520-5.

467a   **Kalter, S. S.** *Viral and immunological diseases in non-human primates.* New York: Alan R. Liss, 1983. (265 pp.) ISBN 0-8451-3401-9.

468   **Kristensen, F.** and **Antczak, D. F.** (Eds). *Advances in veterinary immunology.* New York: Elsevier North-Holland, 1982. (282 pp.) ISBN 0-444-42051-7.

469   **von Muiswinkel, W. B.** and **Cooper, E. L.** (Eds). *Immunology and immunization of fish.* New York: Pergamon Press, 1981. (255 pp.) ISBN 0-08-028831-6.

470   **Tizard, I.** *An introduction to veterinary immunology.* 2nd edn. Philadelphia: W. B. Saunders, 1982. (363 pp.) ISBN 0-7126-8882-9.

Miscellaneous

471 **Daynes, R. A., Spikes, J. D.** and **Krueger, G.** (Eds). *Experimental and clinical photoimmunology.* 2 vols. Boca Raton, Florida: CRC Press, 1983. Vol. 1 (242 pp.) ISBN 0-8493-5370-X. Vol. 2 (208 pp.) ISBN 0-8493-5371-8.

472 **Georgiev, V.** (Ed.). *Survey of drug research in immunologic disease.* Basel: S. Karger. Vol. 1, *Aliphatic derivatives,* 1983 (552 pp.) ISBN 3-8055-3503-1. Vol. 2, *Non-condensed aromatic derivatives,* Part I, 1983 (668 pp.) ISBN 3-8055-3566-X. Vol. 3, *Non-condensed aromatic derivatives,* Part II, 1983 (600 pp.) ISBN 3-8055-3687-9. Vols 4–8, *Non-condensed aromatic derivatives,* Parts III–VII in preparation.

472a **Gibson, G. G., Hubbard, R.** and **Parker, D. V.** *Immunotoxicology.* New York: Academic Press, 1983. (532 pp.) ISBN 0-12-282180-7.

472b **Isojima, S.** and **Billington, W. D.** (Eds). *Reproductive immunology, 1983.* Amsterdam: Elsevier, 1983. (286 pp.) ISBN 0-444-80551-6.

473 **Jones, W. R.** *Immunological fertility regulation.* Oxford: Blackwell Scientific Publications, 1983. (284 pp.) ISBN 0-86793-008-X.

474 **Jones, W. R.** and **Need, J. A.** *Clinical reproductive immunology.* Oxford: Blackwell Scientific Publications, 1984. (320 pp.) ISBN 0-86793-136-1.

475 **Parrish, J. A., Kripke, M. L.** and **Morison, W. L.** (Eds). *Photo-immunology.* Oxford: Blackwell Scientific Publications, 1981. (500 pp.)

476 **Soothill, J. F., Hayward, A. R.** and **Wood, M. B.** (Eds). *Paediatric immunology.* Oxford: Blackwell Scientific Publications, 1981. (500 pp.) ISBN 0-632-00724-9.

477 **Wegmann, T. G.** and **Gill, T. J.** (Eds). *Reproductive immunology.* Oxford: Oxford University Press, 1984. (500 pp.) ISBN 0-19-503096-6.

Indexes to Dissertations (*see* section 5.4)

478 *American Doctoral Dissertations.* Ann Arbor, Michigan: University Microfilms International, 1934–. Annual.

479 *Abstracts of Theses.* London: Aslib, 1978–. Semi-annual. Microfiche only.

480 *British Reports, Translations and Theses.* Boston Spa, West Yorkshire: British Library Lending Division, 1971–. Monthly. ISSN 0144-7556.

481 *Comprehensive Dissertations Index.* Ann Arbor, Michigan: University Microfilms International, 1973–. Annual.

482 *Dissertation Abstracts International:* Section B, *The Sciences and Engineering.* Ann Arbor, Michigan: University Microfilms International, 1938–. Monthly. ISSN 0419-4217.

483 *Dissertation Abstracts International:* Section C, *European Abstracts.* Ann Arbor, Michigan: University Microfilms International, 1976–. Quarterly.

484 *Dissertation Abstracts Online.* Ann Arbor, Michigan: University Microfilms International, 1861–. Updates monthly. *Host:* DIALOG.

485   *Index to theses*. London: Aslib, 1950–. Semi-annual. ISSN 0073-6066.

486   *Masters Abstracts*. Ann Arbor, Michigan: University Microfilms International, 1962–. Quarterly. ISSN 0025-5106.

PATENTS

487   **Crafts-Lighty, A.** *Information sources in biotechnology*. Basingstoke: Macmillan, 1983. (320 pp.) ISBN 0-333-36178-4.

488   **Crespi, R. S.** *Patenting in the biological sciences*. Chichester: John Wiley & Sons, 1982. (211 pp.) ISBN 0-471-10151-6.

489   *Patent Licensing: a Guide to the Literature*. London: Science Reference Library, 1982. (8 pp.) ISSN 0306-4298.

Sources of Patents *(see* section 5.5)

490   *Inpadoc*. McLean, Virginia: Pergamon, 1968–. Weekly updates. *Host:* Pergamon Infoline.

491   *Patsearch*. McLean, Virginia: Pergamon, 1971–. Weekly updates. *Host:* Pergamon Infoline.

REFERENCE WORKS *(see* section 5.6)

Guides to the Literature

492   **Chen, Ching-Chih.** *Health sciences information sources*. Cambridge, Massachusetts: MIT Press, 1981. ISBN 0-262-03074-8.

493   **Crafts-Lighty, A.** *Information sources in biotechnology*. Basingstoke: Macmillan, 1983. (320 pp.) ISBN 0-333-36178-4.

494   **Lilley, G. P.** (Ed.). *Information sources in agriculture and food science*. London: Butterworths, 1981. (603 pp.) ISBN 0-408-10612-3.

495   **Morton, L. T.** and **Godbolt, S.** *Information sources in the medical sciences*. London: Butterworths, 1984. (534 pp.) ISBN 0-408-11473-8.

496   **U.S. National Cancer Institute.** *Directory of cancer research information resources*. 2nd edn. Bethesda, Maryland: U.S. National Cancer Institute, 1979. (250 pp.)

Reference Books

497   *The allergy encyclopedia*. (Edited by the Asthma and Allergy Foundation of America and C. T. Norbach.) St Louis: C. V. Mosby, 1981. (256 pp.) ISBN 0-452-25345-4.

498   *Basic and clinical immunology*. 4th edn. (By D. P. Stites, J. D. Stobo, H. H. Fudenberg and J. V. Wells.) Los Altos, California: Lange Medical Publications, 1982. (775 pp.) ISBN 0-87041-223-X.

499   *Biotechnology made simple: a glossary of recombinant DNA and hybridoma technology*. Richmond: PJB Publications, 1983. (117 pp.)

500 *Black's medical dictionary.* 33rd edn. (Edited by W. A. R. Thompson.) London: A. & C. Black, 1981. (982 pp.) ISBN 0-7136-2128-1.

501 *Butterworth's medical dictionary.* 2nd edn. (Edited by M. Critchley.) London: Butterworths, 1980. ISBN 0-407-00061-5.

501a *Compendium of immunology.* 2nd edn. (Edited by L. M. Schwartz.) Wokingham: Van Nostrand Reinhold, 1980. (515 pp.) ISBN 0-442-27472-6.

502 *A dictionary of immunology.* (Edited by W. J. Herbert, P. C. Wilkinson and D. I. Stott.) Oxford: Blackwell Scientific Publications, 1984. (250 pp.) ISBN 0-632-00984-5.

503 *Dictionary of microbiology.* (By P. Singleton and D. Sainsbury.) Chichester: Wiley Interscience, 1981. (490 pp.) ISBN 0-471-99658-0.

504 *A dictionary of virology.* (Edited by K. E. K. Rowson, T. A. L. Rees and B. W. J. Mahy.) Oxford: Blackwell Scientific Publications, 1981. (230 pp.) ISBN 0-632-00784-2.

505 *Encyclopaedia Britannica.* Chicago: Encyclopaedia Britannica, 1975. ISBN 0-85229-297-X.

506 *Encyclopedia of clinical assessment.* (Edited by R. H. Woody.) 2 vols. San Francisco: Jassey-Bass, 1980. ISBN 0-87589-446-1.

507 *Glossary of haematological and serological terms.* (By P. Samson.) London: Butterworths, 1973. (128 pp.) ISBN 0-407-72720-5.

508 *Glossary of immunological terms.* (By W. J. Halliday.) London: Butterworths, 1971. (96 pp.) ISBN 0-407-72740-X.

509 *Handbook of experimental immunology.* 3rd edn. Vol. 3. (Edited by D. M. Weir.) Oxford: Blackwell Scientific Publications, 1978. ISBN 0-632-00186-0.

510 *Inverted medical dictionary.* (Edited by W. A. Rigal.) Westport, Connecticut: Technomic, 1976. ISBN 0-87762-170-5.

511 *McGraw-Hill encyclopedia of science and technology.* 5th edn. New York: McGraw-Hill, 1982.

512 *Practical immunology.* 2nd edn. (By L. Hudson and F. ʹC. May). Oxford: Blackwell Scientific Publications, 1980. (359 pp.) ISBN 0-632-00353-7.

512a *Saunders' dictionary and encyclopedia of laboratory medicine.* (By J. L. Bennington.) Philadelphia: W. B. Saunders, 1983. (1674 pp.) ISBN 0-7216-1714-X.

513 *Stedman's medical dictionary.* 24th edn. Baltimore: Williams & Wilkins, 1982. (1678 pp.) ISBN 0-683-07915-8.

514 *Van Nostrand's scientific encyclopedia.* 6th edn. (Edited by D. M. Considine.) New York: Van Nostrand, 1983. (3100 pp.) ISBN 0-442-25161-0.

Biographical Reference Works

515 *American men and women of science: physical and biological sciences.* New York: Jaques Cattell Press (Bowker), 1906–. Irregular. ISSN 0065-9347. *Host:* DIALOG.

516 *Biographical memoirs of the National Academy of Sciences.* Washington, D.C.: National Academy of Sciences, 1953–. Irregular.

517 *Biographical Memoirs of Fellows of the Royal Society.* London: Royal Society of London, 1955–. Annual. ISSN 0080-4606.

518 *Federation of American Societies for Experimental Biology: Directory of Members.* Bethesda, Maryland: The Federation. Annual.

519 *International medical who's who.* Harlow, Essex: Longman, 1983. Irregular. ISBN 0-582-90102-2; 0-582-90103-0.

520 *Marquis Who's Who.* Chicago: Marquis Who's Who, Current. Updated quarterly. *Host:* DIALOG.

521 *Who was who.* London: A. & C. Black, 1967–81.

    Vol. 1, 1897–1915. ISBN 0-7136-0168-X

    Vol. 2, 1916–1928. ISBN 0-7136-0169-8

    Vol. 3, 1929–1940. ISBN 0-7136-0170-1

    Vol. 4, 1941–1950. ISBN 0-7136-0171-X

    Vol. 5, 1951–1960. ISBN 0-7136-0172-8

    Vol. 6, 1961–1970. ISBN 0-7136-2008-0

    Vol. 7, 1971–1980. ISBN 0-7136-2176-1

also index 1897–1980. ISBN 0-7136-2177-X.

522 *Who's Who.* A. & C. Black, 1849–. Annual. ISSN 0083-937X.

523 *Who's who in British scientists 1980/81.* 3rd edn. London: Simon Books, 1980. ISBN 0-86229-001-5.

CLASSIFICATION SCHEMES *(see* section 5.8)

524 **Barnard, C.** *A classification for medical and veterinary libraries.* London: H. K. Lewis, 1955. (179 pp.)

525 *Bliss bibliographic classification.* 2nd edn. (Edited by J. Mills and V. Broughton.) London: Butterworths, 1980. ISBN 0-408-7082-X.

526 *Dewey decimal classification.* 19th edn. Albany, New York: Forest Press, 1979. 3 vols. (2692 pp.) ISBN 0-910608-23-7.

527 *Library of Congress classification. Class Q, Science.* 6th edn. Washington, D.C.: Library of Congress, 1973. (415 pp.) ISBN 0-8444-0075-0.

528 *National Library of Medicine classification.* 4th edn. Bethesda, Maryland: National Library of Medicine, 1978. (286 pp.)

529 *Universal decimal classification: biological sciences.* 2nd edn. London: British Standards Institution, 1979.

Part III

DIRECTORY OF ORGANIZATIONS AND DATABASE HOSTS

DIRECTORY OF ORGANIZATIONS AND DATABASE HOSTS

INTERNATIONAL UNION OF IMMUNOLOGICAL SOCIETIES (IUIS)

Officers

530 President: Baruj Benacerraf
Department of Pathology
Harvard Medical School
25 Shattuck Street
Boston, Massachusetts 02215
USA

531 Vice-President: Alain de Weck
Institute of Clinical Immunology
Inselspital
CH-3010 Berne
Switzerland

532 Secretary-General: Jacob B. Natvig
Institute of Immunology and Rheumatology
Rikshospitalet University Hospital
Fr. Qvamsgt. 1
Oslo 1
Norway

533 Treasurer: Henri Isliker
Université de Lausanne
Institut de Biochimie
Chemin des Bouveresses
CH-1066 Epalinges
Switzerland

534 Past President: Michael Sela
Department of Chemical Immunology
Weizmann Institute of Science
Rehovot
Israel

Committees

535   Education Committee
Secretary: Franco Celada
Laboratory of Cell Biology
Via G. Romagnosi 18
I-00196 Roma
Italy

536   Nomenclature Committee
Secretary: I. Tizard
Department of Veterinary Microbiology and Immunology
University of Guelph
Guelph, Ontario
Canada N1G 2W1

537   Standardization Committee
Chairman: R. E. Ritts, Jr
Mayo Foundation Clinic
Rochester, Minnesota 55905
USA

538   Symposium Committee
Chairman: H. Metzger
American Association of Immunologists
9650 Rockville Pike
Bethesda, Maryland 20814
USA

539   Clinical Immunology Committee
Secretary: Dr W. Knapp
Institute of Immunology
Borschkegasse 8
A-1090 Vienna
Austria

540   Veterinary Immunology Committee
Secretary: F. Kristensen
Institut für Klinische Immunologie
Inselspital
CH-3010 Berne
Switzerland

541   Publication Committee
Chairman: Göran Möller
Karolinska Institute
Department of Immunobiology
Wallenberg Laboratory
Lilla Frescati
S-104 05 Stockholm 50
Sweden

542   European Federation
       Secretary-General: J. D. Naysmith
       Department of Pathology
       University Medical School
       University Walk
       Bristol BS8 1TD
       England

NATIONAL SOCIETIES OF IMMUNOLOGY AFFILIATED TO IUIS

543   **Argentina**
       (Sociedad Argentina de Immunología)
       L. Rumi
       Instituto de Medicino y Biologici Experimental
       Obligado 2490
       1428 Buenos Aires

544   **Australia**
       (Australian Society for Immunology)
       S. J. Prowse
       Department of Immunology
       The John Curtin School of Medical Research
       Australian National University
       P.O. Box 334
       Canberra City, ACT 2601

545   **Austria**
       (Österreichische Gesellschaft für Allergologie und Immunologie)
       W. Knapp
       Institute of Immunology
       University of Vienna
       Borschkegasse 8a
       A-1090 Vienna

546   **Belgium**
       (Belgian Immunology Society)
       B. Van Camp
       A.Z.–V.U.B.
       Dienst Immunologie–Hematologie
       101 Laarbeeklaan
       B-1090 Bruxelles
       Belgium

547   **Brazil**
       (Sociedade Brasiliera de Immunologia)
       W. Dias da Silva
       Instituto de Ciências Biomédicas da USP
       Departemento de Microbiologia e Imunologia, Ed Didática
       Biomédicas II (S32)
       00508 — Cid. Universitária
       São Paulo — SP.

548 **Bulgaria**
(Bulgarian Society for Immunology)
S. Trifonov
Institute of General and Comparative Pathology
Bulgarian Academy of Sciences
G. Bonchev Str., Blok 3
1113 Sofia

549 **Canada**
(Canadian Society for Immunology)
A. Froese
Department of Immunology
University of Manitoba
730 William Avenue
Winnipeg, Manitoba R3E 0W3

550 **Chile**
(Sociedad Chilena de Inmunología)
E. Jurlow
Sociedad Chilena de Inmunología
Casilla 15179
Santiago 11

551 **France**
(Société Française d'Immunologie)
P. Burtin
Centre National de la Recherche Scientifique sur le Cancer
Boîte Postal n° 8
F-94800 Villejuif

552 **German Democratic Republic**
(Gesellschaft für Klinische und Experimentelle Immunologie der DDR)
J. Kaden
Städtisches Krankenhaus im Friedrichshain
Urologische Klinik
Leninallee 49
1017 Berlin

553 **Federal Republic of Germany**
(Gesellschaft für Immunologie)
H. G. Schwick
Behringwerke AG
D-3550 Marburg/Lahn

554 **Greece**
(Greek Society of Immunology)
V. Syripoulu
Greek Society of Immunology
4 Papadiamantopoyloy Str
Athens

555 **Hungary**
(Hungarian Society for Immunology)
G. Gy. Petrányi
National Institute of Haematology and Blood Transfusion
P.O. Box 44
1502 Budapest

556 **India**
(Indian Immunology Society)
A. N. Malaviya
Indian Immunology Society
Clinical Immunology Service
Department of Medicine
All India Institute of Medical Sciences
Ansari Nagar, New Delhi 110 016

557 **Israel**
(Israel Immunology Society)
I. R. Cohen
Department of Cell Biology
Weizmann Institute of Science
Rehovot

558 **Italy**
(Societa Italiana di Immunologia ed Immunopatologia)
A. Carbonara
Istituto di Genetica Medica — Universita
Via Santena 19
I-10126 Torino

559 **Japan**
(Japanese Society for Immunology)
M. Hanaoka
Department of Pathology
Institute for Virus Research
Kyoto University
Shogoin Kawaramachi
Sakyo-ku
Kyoto 606

560 **Mexico**
(Sociedad Mexicana de Inmunología)
K. Willms
Sociedad Mexicana de Inmunologia
Apartado Postal No. 70228
Mexico 20, D.F.

561 **Netherlands**
(Vereniging voor Immunologie)
P. J. A. Capel
Department of Nephrology
Academy Hospital
St Radboudziekenhuis

P.O. Box 9101
NL-6500 HB Nijmegen
The Netherlands

562 **Nigeria**
(Nigeria Society for Immunology)
M. Ola. Ojo
Department of Veterinary Microbiology and Parasitology
University of Ibadan
Ibadan

563 **Poland**
(Polish Immunological Society)
J. Zeromski
Polish Society for Immunology
Department of Immunology and Rheumatology
ul. Szkolna 8/12
60-067 Poznan

564 **Portugal**
(Sociedade Portuguesa de Imunologia)
A. de Freitas
Departemento de Imunologia
Faculdade de Ciências Medicas
Campo de Santana 130
1 198 Lisboa, Portugal

565 **Romania**
(Romanian Commission of Immunology)
A. Sulica
Department of Immunology
Victor Babes Institute
Spl. Independentei 99–101
Bucharest 76201

566 **Scandinavia**
(Scandinavian Society for Immunology)
H. Bennich
BMC
P.O. Box 575
S-751 23 Uppsala
Sweden

567 **Spain**
(Sociedad Española de Inmunología)
M. Ortiz de Landazuri
Plaza de Santa Barbara 4
Madrid 4

568 **Switzerland**
(Schweizerische Gesellschaft für Allergie und Immunologie)
B. Wütrich
Universitatsspital Zürich
Dermatologische Klinik
Allergiestation
CH-8091 Zürich

569 **Turkey**
(Turkish Society for Immunology)
O. Ilter
Cocuk Hastaliklari Klinigi Cerrahpasa Hastanesi
Aksaray — Istanbul

570 **United Kingdom**
(British Society for Immunology)
A. R. Sanderson
BSI Secretariat
P.O. Box 35
East Grinstead
West Sussex RH19 3UT

571 **USA**
(American Association of Immunologists)
H. Metzger
9650 Rockville Pike
Bethesda, Maryland 20014

572 **Venezuela**
(Sociedad Venezolana de Alergía e Inmunología)
F. Ortega
Sociedad Venezolana de Alergía e Inmunología
Apartado No. 68.937
(Altamira)
Caracas 106

573 **Yugoslavia**
(Yugoslav Immunological Society)
V. Kotnik
Institute of Microbiology
Zaloska 4
61104 Ljubljana

Societies Admitted Recently

574 **China**
Wu an Jan, Deputy Head,
Department of Immunology
Institute of Basic Medical Science
Chinese Academy of Medical Science
Beijing, People's Republic of China

575 **Taiwan**
Tsong-Chou Lynn
Society of Immunology located at Taipei
National Taiwan University Hospital
Chanc-te Street, Taipei

Affiliated Commission

576 **International Society of Immunopharmacology**
L. Chedid
Immunothérapie Expérimentale
Institut Pasteur
28 rue du Dr Roux
F-75724 Paris Cedex 15
France

ADDRESSES OF SELECTED ORGANIZATIONS

International

577 Collegium Internationale Allergologicum
c/o Professor A. De Weck
Institute for Clinical Immunology
Inselspital
CH-3010 Berne
Switzerland

578 European Academy of Allergology and Clinical Immunology
Scientific Secretariat
I Clinica Medica
Policlinico Umberto
I-00161 Rome
Italy

579 European Committee for Clinical Laboratory Standards
ECCLS Central Office
c/o Wellcome Research Laboratory
Langley Court
Beckenham
Kent BR3 3BS
England

580 European Federation of Immunological Societies, *see* IUIS

581 European Molecular Biology Organization
Postfach 10 22 40
69 Heidelberg
Federal Republic of Germany

582 International Association of Allergology
1390 Sherbrooke Street West
Montreal
Quebec H3G 1K2
Canada

583   International Association of Biological Standardization
      Biostandards
      Case postale 25
      CH-1231 Conches-Genève
      Switzerland

584   International Council of Scientific Unions
      51 Blvd de Montmorency
      F-75016 Paris
      France

585   International Society of Developmental and Comparative Immunology
      c/o Dr R. K. Wright
      Department of Anatomy
      School of Medicine
      University of California
      Los Angeles, California 90024
      USA

586   Reticulo-endothelial Society
      c/o Dr Sherwood M. Reichard
      Medical College of Georgia
      Augusta, Georgia 30912
      USA

587   Transplantation Society
      Department of Surgery
      Health Sciences Center
      T-19
      RM040
      State University of Stony Brook
      Stony Brook
      New York 11794
      USA

588   Immunology Unit
      World Health Organization
      Avenue Appia
      CH-1211 Geneva 27
      Switzerland

589   World Association of Veterinary Microbiologists, Immunologists and
      Specialists in Infectious Diseases (WAVMI)
      c/o W.J. Penhale
      School of Veterinary Studies
      Murdoch
      W. Australia 6150

WHO Collaborating Centres in Immunology (Figures in parentheses indicate number of centres designated within the same institute)

590   Walter and Eliza Hall Institute of Medical Research
      Melbourne University
      Victoria
      Australia (3)

591   Instituto Butantan
      São Paulo
      Brazil

592   Division of Clinical Immunology and Allergy
      Montreal General Hospital
      Montreal
      Canada

593   Department of Immunology
      Institute of Microbiology
      Prague
      Czechoslovakia

594   Centre Départemental de Transfusion Sanguine et de Génétique Humaine
      Bois-Guillaume
      Seine-Maritime
      France

595   Laboratoire d'Immunochimie
      Institut de Recherches Scientifiques sur le Cancer
      Centre National de la Recherche Scientifique
      Villejuif
      Val-de-Marne
      France

596   Department of Biochemistry
      All India Institute of Medical Sciences
      Indian Council of Medical Research
      New Delhi
      India

597   Department of Chemical Immunology and Cell Biology
      Weizmann Institute of Science
      Rehovot
      Israel

598   Department of Biochemistry,
      Faculty of Medicine
      Hokkaido University
      Sapporo
      Japan

599   Faculty of Medicine
      University of Nairobi
      Kenya

600   School of Medicine
      American University of Beirut
      Lebanon

601   Children's Hospital of Mexico
      Mexico City
      Mexico

602 Department of Chemical Pathology
University College Hospital
Ibadan
Nigeria

603 Faculty of Medicine
University of Singapore
Singapore

604 Department of Medical Microbiology
University of Lund
Sweden

605 Basle Institute of Immunology
Basle
Switzerland

606 Institut de Biochimie
University of Lausanne
Switzerland (3)

607 Gamaleja Institute of Epidemiology and Microbiology
Moscow
USSR (3)

608 Chester Beatty Research Institute
Institute of Cancer Research
Royal Cancer Hospital
London
England

609 Department of Immunology
Middlesex Hospital Medical School
London
England

610 Department of Immunology
Royal Postgraduate Medical School
University of London
England

611 Medical Research Council's Blood Group Reference Laboratory
London
England

612 Department of Immunology
City of Hope National Medical Center
Duarte
California
USA

613 National Cancer Institute
National Institutes of Health
Bethesda
Maryland
USA (2)

614   Center for Immunology
      School of Medicine
      State University of New York at Buffalo
      New York
      USA

615   Roswell Park Memorial Institute
      New York State Department of Health
      Buffalo
      New York
      USA

616   Department of Biology
      Western Reserve University
      Cleveland
      Ohio
      USA

617   Department of Molecular Immunology
      Scripps Clinic and Research Foundation
      La Jolla
      California
      USA

Commercial Organizations

618   Amersham International plc
      Amersham HP7 9LL
      England

619   Boehringer Mannheim Biochemicals
      7941 Castleway Drive
      P.O. Box 50816
      Indianapolis
      Indiana 46250
      USA

620   Celltech
      244 Bath Road
      Slough
      Berkshire SL1 4DY
      England

621   Cetus Immune Corporation
      3400 West Bayshore Road
      Palo Alto
      California 94303
      USA

622   Dynatech Laboratories Ltd
      Daux Road
      Billinghurst
      Sussex
      England

623 Flow Laboratories
     P.O. Box 17
     Irvine
     Ayrshire KA12 8NB
     Scotland

624 Gibco Europe Ltd
     P.O. Box 35
     3 Washington Road
     Paisley PA3 4EP
     Scotland

625 Glaxo Group Research Limited
     Ware
     Hertfordshire SG12 0DB
     England

626 ICI — Corporate Biosciences Group
     Molecular Genetics Section
     The Heath
     Runcorn
     England

627 ICI plc
     Pharmaceuticals Division
     Mereside Research Laboratory
     Alderley Park
     Macclesfield
     Cheshire SK10 4TG
     England

628 Lilly Research Centre Ltd
     Erl Wood Manor
     London Road
     Windlesham
     Surrey GU20 6PH
     England

629 LKB
     232 Addington Road
     South Croydon
     Surrey CR2 8YD
     England

630 May and Baker Limited
     Rainham Road South
     Dagenham
     Essex RM10 7XS
     England

631 Merck, Sharp & Dohme
     Hertford Road
     Hoddesden
     Hertfordshire EN11 9BU
     England

632   MRC Laboratory Animals Centre
      Carshalton
      Surrey
      England

633   New England Nuclear GmbH
      Postfach 40 12 40
      Dreieich
      Federal Republic of Germany
      also: 2453 46th Ave., Lachine, Quebec H8T 3C9, Canada
      also: 549 Albany Street, Boston, Massachusetts 02118, USA

634   Medix — OY Medix AB
      PB 819
      SF-00101 Helsinki 10
      Finland

635   Nordic Immunological Laboratories
      P.O. Box 22
      NL-5000 AA Tilburg
      The Netherlands

636   Pharmacia Fine Chemicals
      Box 175
      S-751 04 Uppsala 1
      Sweden

637   Roche Products
      P.O. Box 8
      Welwyn Garden City
      Hertfordshire AL7 3AY
      England

638   Sandoz Research Institute
      Brunner Strasse 59
      A-1235 Vienna
      Austria

639   Serotec Ltd
      Station Road
      Blackthorn
      Bicester
      Oxford OX6 0TP
      England

640   Sigma Chemical Company
      Fancy Road
      Poole
      Dorset BH17 7NH
      England

641   Smith Klein Corporation
      Research Institute
      The Frythe
      Welwyn
      Hertfordshire
      England

642   Tago Inc.
      Immunodiagnostic Reagents
      1 Edwards Court
      Burlingame
      California 94010
      USA

643   UCB — Bioproducts SA
      rue Berkendael, 68
      B-1060 Bruxelles
      Belgium

644   Wellcome Diagnostics
      Temple Hill
      Dartford DA1 5AH
      England

645   Wellcome Research Laboratories
      Langley Court
      Beckenham
      Kent BR3 3BS
      England

UK — Societies

646   British Society for Allergy and Clinical Immunology (BSACI)
      c/o Chest Department
      St Bartholomew's Hospital
      West Smithfield
      London EC1A 7BE

647   British Transplantation Society
      Guy's Hospital
      London SE1 9RT

648   Immunocytochemistry Club
      Royal Postgraduate Medical School
      Hammersmith Hospital
      Ducane Road
      London W12 0HS

649   Interferon Club
      A. Morris
      Biological Science Department
      University of Warwick
      Coventry CV4 7AL

650   Metchnikoff Club (The Edinburgh Immunology Group)
       Dr K. James
       Department of Surgery
       University of Edinburgh Medical School
       Teviot Place
       Edinburgh EH8 9AG

651   Royal College of Pathologists
       2 Carlton Terrace
       London SW1 5AF

652   Royal Society of Medicine
       1 Wimpole Street
       London W1M 8AE

653   Society for General Microbiology
       Harvest House
       62 London Road
       Reading
       Berkshire RG1 5AS

654   West Yorkshire Immunology Group
       Dr A. H. Balfour
       Regional Public Health Laboratory
       Bridle Path Road
       Leeds LS15 7TR

UK — Government

Agricultural and Food Research Council

655   Meat Research Institute
       Langford
       Bristol BS18 7DY

656   Institute of Animal Physiology
       Babraham
       Cambridge CB2 4AT

657   Institute for Research on Animal Diseases
       Compton
       Newbury
       Berkshire RG16 0NN

658   Moredun Institute (ADRA)
       408 Gilmerton Road
       Edinburgh EH17 7JH

659   Animal Virus Research Institute
       Pirbright
       Woking
       Surrey GU24 0NF

Medical Research Council

660 Laboratory of Molecular Biology
Hills Road
Cambridge CB2 2QH

661 Clinical Research Centre
Watford Road
Harrow HA1 3UJ

662 National Institute for Medical Research
Mill Hill
London NW7 1AA

National Biological Standards Board UK

663 National Institute for Biological Standards and Control
Holly Hill
Hampstead
London NW3 6RB

Public Health Laboratory Service

664 Central Public Health Laboratory
Colindale Avenue
London NW9 5HT

665 Communicable Disease Surveillance Centre
61 Colindale Avenue
London NW9 5EQ

666 Centre for Applied Microbiology and Research
Porton Down
Salisbury
Wiltshire SP4 0JG

UK — Private Research Institutes

667 Beatson Institute for Cancer Research
Garscube Estate
Bearsden
Glasgow G61 1BD

668 Cancer Research Campaign
2 Carlton House Terrace
London SW1Y 5AR

669 Imperial Cancer Research Fund
Lincoln's Inn Fields
London WC2A 3PX

670 Institute of Cancer Research
Chester Beatty Research Institute
237 Fulham Road
London SW3 6JB

671   Paterson Laboratories
      Wilmslow Road
      Manchester M20 9BX

UK — Universities and Colleges

672   University College of Wales
      Aberystwyth
      Dyfed SY23 2AX

673   Department of Immunology
      The Medical School
      Birmingham B15 2TJ

674   Immunobiology Group
      The University
      Bristol BS8 1TH

675   Division of Immunology
      Department of Pathology
      Addenbrooke's Hospital
      Hills Road
      Cambridge CB2 2QQ

676   North East Surrey College of Technology
      Reigate Road
      Ewell
      Surrey KT17 3DS

677   Department of Bacteriology and Immunology
      Western Infirmary
      Glasgow University
      Glasgow G11 6NT

678   Department of Allergy and Clinical Immunology
      Cardiothoracic Institute
      Brompton Hospital
      London SW3 6HP

679   Chelsea College
      University of London
      Manresa Road
      London SW3 6LX

680   Department of Immunology
      Institute of Child Health
      London University
      30 Guildford Street
      London WC1N 1EH

681   Department of Immunology and Liver Unit
      King's College Hospital Medical School
      Denmark Hill
      London SE5 8RX

682   Bone and Joint Research Unit
      London Hospital Medical College
      Turner Street
      London E1 2AD

683   Immunology Unit
      Department of Medical Microbiology
      London School of Hygiene and Tropical Medicine
      London WC1E 7HT

684   Department of Immunology
      Middlesex Hospital Medical School
      London W1P 9PG

685   Department of Immunology
      St Mary's Hospital Medical School
      Praed Street
      London W2 1PG

686   Departments of Immunology and Haematology
      St Thomas's Hospital Medical School
      London SE1 7EH

687   Division of Biochemistry
      North East London Polytechnic
      Romford Road
      London E15 4LZ

688   Royal Postgraduate Medical School
      (University of London)
      150 Ducane Road
      London W12 0HS

689   Imperial Cancer Research Fund
      Tumour Immunology Unit
      Department of Zoology
      University College London
      Gower Street
      London WC1E 6BT

690   Department of Clinical Rheumatism
      Hope Hospital
      Manchester M6 8HD

691   Department of Immunology and Rheumatism Research Centre
      Medical School
      University of Manchester
      Oxford Road
      Manchester M13 9PL

692   University of Nottingham
      University Park
      Nottingham NG7 2RD

693   MRC Immunology Unit
      Sir William Dunn School of Pathology
      Oxford

694   Nuffield Department of Medicine
       John Radcliffe Hospital
       Headington
       Oxford OX3 9DU

695   Department of Haematology
       University of Sheffield
       Royal Hallamshire Hospital
       Glossop Road
       Sheffield S10 2JF

696   Department of Immunochemistry
       Tenovus Research Laboratory
       University of Southampton
       General Hospital
       Southampton SO9 4XX

697   Brunel University
       Uxbridge
       Middlesex UB8 3PH

USA — Societies

American Academy of Allergy (AAA)

698   American Association for Clinical Immunology and Allergy
       P.O. Box 912
       DTS
       Omaha
       Nebraska 68101

699   American Association for Tissue Banks
       1211 Parklawn Drive
       Rockville
       Maryland 20852

700   American Board of Clinical Immunology and Allergy
       P.O. Box 912
       Omaha
       Nebraska 68101

701   American Board of Allergy and Immunology
       University City Science Center
       3624 Market Street
       Philadelphia
       Pennsylvania 19104

702   American Dermatological Society of Allergy and Immunology
       University of Missouri Medical Center
       MIF3 807 Stadium Road
       Columbia
       Missouri 65212

702a American Society for Histocompatibility and Immunogenetics
211 East 43rd Street
New York 10017

703 Federation of American Societies for Experimental Biology
9650 Rockville Pike
Bethesda
Maryland 20014

704 Foundation for Cure
12 Oriole Lane
Oceanside
California 92054

USA — Government

705 National Cancer Institute
National Institutes of Health
Bethesda
Maryland 20205

706 Arthritis Branch
National Institute of Arthritis, Diabetes, Digestive and Kidney Diseases
Bethesda
Maryland 20205

707 National Institutes of Health
Bethesda
Maryland 20014

708 National Institute of Child Health and Human Development
Bethesda
Maryland 20205

709 Neuroimmunology Branch
National Institute of Neurological and Communicative Disorders and
    Stroke
Bethesda
Maryland 20205

710 Laboratories of Immunology and Microbial Immunity
National Institute of Allergy and Infectious Diseases
National Institutes of Health
Bethesda
Maryland 20205

USA — Private Research Institutes

711 Dana Farber Cancer Institute
Boston
Massachusetts 02115

712 Sidney Farber Cancer Institute
Boston
Massachusetts 02115

713   Massachusetts Institute of Technology
       Cambridge
       Massachusetts 02139

714   Howard Hughes Medical Institute Laboratories
       University of California
       San Francisco
       California 94143

715   Mayo Foundation Clinic
       Rochester
       Minnesota 55905

716   Michigan Cancer Foundation
       Detroit
       Michigan 48201

717   The Molecular Biology Institute
       UCLA School of Medicine
       Los Angeles
       California 90024

718   Palo Alto Medical Foundation
       Palo Alto
       California 94301

719   The Salk Institute of Biological Studies
       San Diego
       California 92138

720   The Scripps Clinic and Research Foundation
       10666 North Torrey Pines Road
       La Jolla
       California 92037

721   The Wistar Institute
       136th and Spruce Streets
       Philadelphia
       Pennsylvania 19104

USA — Universities

722   Cellular Immunobiology Unit of the Tumour Institute
       University of Alabama in Birmingham
       Birmingham
       Alabama 35294

723   University of California School of Medicine at Davis
       Davis
       California 95616

724   University of California
       San Diego
       La Jolla
       California 92093

725 University of California at San Francisco
     California 94143

726 Departments of Pathology and Biochemistry and the Committee of
         Immunology
     University of Chicago
     Chicago
     Illinois 60637

727 Columbia University College of Physicians and Surgeons
     New York 10027

728 University of Colorado Health Science Center
     Denver
     Colorado

729 Division of Immunology
     Duke University Medical Center
     Durham
     North Carolina 27710

730 North Western University Medical School
     Evanston
     Illinois 60201

731 Department of Pathology
     Harvard Medical School
     25 Shattuck Street
     Boston
     Massachusetts 02215

732 Johns Hopkins University School of Medicine
     Baltimore
     Maryland 21205

733 University of Michigan Medical School
     Ann Arbor
     Michigan 48109

734 Departments of Medicine and Microbiology
     State University of New York at Buffalo
     Buffalo
     New York 14215

735 School of Medicine
     University of Pennsylvania
     Philadelphia
     Pennsylvania 19104

736 The Rockefeller University
     New York
     New York 10021

737 Department of Pathology
     Stanford University of Medicine
     Stanford
     California 94305

738   University of Texas Health Centre at Dallas
       5323 Harry Hines Boulevard
       Dallas
       Texas 75235

739   University of Washington
       Seattle
       Washington 98104

740   Yale University School of Medicine
       333 Cedar Street
       New Haven
       Connecticut 06510

Australia

741   Australian Monoclonal Development
       65 Dickson Street
       Artarmon 2064
       New South Wales

742   Department of Immunology
       The John Curtin School of Medical Research
       Australian National University
       Canberra
       ACT 2601

743   The Walter and Eliza Hall Institute of Medical Research
       Royal Melbourne Hospital
       Melbourne
       Victoria 3050

744   CSIRO Molecular and Cellular Biology Unit
       Genetics Research Laboratory
       Delhi Road
       North Ryde
       New South Wales 2113

745   National Biological Standards Laboratory
       Private Bag No. 7
       Parkville
       Victoria 3052

746   Immunology Unit
       Medical Research Department
       Kanematsu Memorial Institute
       Sydney Hospital
       Sydney

747   Ludwig Institute for Cancer Research
       University of Sydney
       Sydney

748   Australian National Animal Health Laboratory
       Postbag 24
       Geelong
       Victoria 3220

749   The Clinical Immunology Research Centre
       University of Sydney
       Sydney
       New South Wales 2006

Austria

750   Institut für Immunologie der Universität Wien
       Borschkegasse 8A
       A-1090 Wien

Canada

751   Department of Immunology
       University of Alberta
       Edmonton
       Alberta T6H 4H7

752   Merck-Frosst Canada Inc.
       Kirkland
       Quebec H9R 4P8

753   Institute Armond Frappier
       531 Boulevard des Prairies
       Laval des Rapides
       Quebec H7V 1B7

754   Institute of Microbiology and Hygiene
       University of Montreal
       Montreal
       Quebec H3C 3J7

755   McGill University
       3640 University Street
       Montreal
       Quebec H3A 2T5

756   Ontario Cancer Institute and Institute of Immunology
       University of Toronto
       Toronto
       Ontario M5S 1A8

757   MRC Group for Allergy Research
       Department of Immunology
       University of Manitoba
       Winnipeg R3E 0W3

France

758   Centre d'Immunologie et de Biologie Parasitaire
       INSERM U167
       Institut Pasteur
       15 rue Comitte Guerin
       F-59019 Lille Cedex

759   Centre d'Immunologie
       INSERM-CNRS
       Marseille-Luminy
       F-13288 Marseille Cedex 9

759a   Laboratoire Immunotech
       Luminy Case 915
       F-13288 Marseille Cedex 9

760   Laboratoire d'Immunopharmacologie des Tumeurs
       Centre Paul Larmarque
       Montpellier

761   Institut Pasteur
       28 rue du Docteur Roux
       F-75724 Paris Cedex 15

761a   Centre d'Immunopathologie et Immunologie Experimentale
       Claude Bernard et INSERM Association
       F-75012 Paris

762   Institut National de la Santé et de la Recherche Médicale
       101 rue de Tolbiac
       F-75645 Paris Cedex 13

763   Laboratoire d'Immunologie et de Virologie des Tumeurs
       INSERM U152
       CNRS ERA 781
       Hôpital Cochin
       F-75674 Paris Cedex 14

764   Centre National de la Recherche Scientifique (CNRS)
       15 Quai Anatole France
       F-75700 Paris

765   Université Pierre et Marie Curie
       Laboratoire d'Immunologie Comparée
       Paris

766   Laboratoire d'Immunochimie et Immunopathologie
       Hôpital St Louis
       2 Place du Dr Fournier
       F-75475 Paris Cedex 10

767   Centre National de la Recherche Scientifique sur le Cancer
       Boite Postal No. 8
       F-94800 Villejuif

768   Société Française d'Allergologie
      1 rue du Val de Grace
      F-75005 Paris

Federal Republic of Germany

769   Lehrstuhl Med. Mikrobiol. Immunol. Arbeitsgruppe Infektabwehrmech
      Ruhr-Universität
      D-4630 Bochum

770   Institut für Genetik
      University of Cologne
      D-5000 Cologne 41

771   Institut für Medizinische Virologie und Immunologie
      Hufelelandstr. 55
      D-4300 Essen

772   Max-Planck-Institut für Immunobiologie
      Postfach 1169
      Stubeweg 51
      D-7800 Freiburg

773   Institute of Clinical Immunology and Blood Transfusion
      University of Giessen
      D-6300 Giessen

774   Institut für Immunologie und Serologie
      Universität Heidelberg
      D-6900 Heidelberg

775   Institut für Immunologie und Genetik
      Deutsches Krebsforschungszentrum
      D-6900 Heidelberg

776   Institute of Molecular Genetics
      Universität Heidelberg
      D-6900 Heidelberg

777   Institut für Med. Mikrobiol.
      Johannes Gutenberg Universität
      D-6500 Mainz

778   Institut für Physiologie
      Universität Marburg
      D-3550 Marburg

779   Department of Immunology
      Universität Munster
      D-4400 Munster

780   Max-Planck-Institut für Biologie
      Abteilung Immunogenetik
      Correnstrasse 42
      D-7400 Tübingen

781   Department of Medicine
      University of Tübingen

782   Immunology Laboratory
      Medizinische Klinik
      D-7400 Tübingen

783   Institute of Virology and Immunobiology
      University of Würzburg
      Versbacher Str.
      D-8700 Würzburg

784   Department of Immunology
      University of Ulm
      P.O. Box 4066
      D-7900 Ulm

Israel

785   Department of Cell Biology
      The Weizmann Institute of Science
      Rehovot 76100

Italy

786   Immunitalia
      Via Castagretta
      I-00040 Pomezia, Roma

787   Istituto di Ricerche Farmacologiche
      Mario Megri
      Milano

788   Laboratory of Immunopharmacology
      Sclavo Research Centre
      Seina

789   Cattedra Immunologia
      Viale Università 37
      I-00161 Roma

790   Università, Milano
      Via F. Sforza, 35
      I-20122 Milano

791   Università, Padova
      Via Gattamelata 64
      I-35128 Padova

Japan

792   Institute for Medical Immunology
      School of Medicine
      Kumamoto University
      2-2-1 Honjo
      Kumamoto 860

793   Osaka University Hospital
      1-1 Yamadaoka
      Suita 565

794   Aichi Cancer Center Research Institute
      Kanokoden
      Tashiro-cho
      Chikusa-ku
      Nagoya 464

795   Department of Immunology
      Faculty of Medicine, University of Tokyo
      7-3-1 Hongo
      Bunkoy-ku
      Tokyo 113

796   Institute for Molecular and Cellular Biology
      Osaka University
      Suita
      Osaka 565

797   Institute of Immunological Science
      Hokkaido University
      Kita 15-jo
      Nishi 7 chome
      Kita-ku
      Sapporo 060

798   Institute of Immunology
      School of Medicine
      Kyoto University
      Yoshida Konoe
      Sakyo-ku
      Kyoto 606

799   National Cancer Center
      5-1-1 Tsukijii
      Chu-o-ku
      Tokyo 104

800   National Institute of Health
      Kamiosaki
      Shinagawa-ku
      Tokyo 141

Netherlands

801   Department of Medicine
      Sint Radboudziekenhuis
      Geert Grootplein Zuid 8
      University of Nijmegen

802   Netherlands Cancer Institute
      Plesmanlaan 121
      NL-1066 CX Amsterdam

803   Immunology Section of the Laboratory of Microbiology
       Medical Faculty
       State University of Utrecht

804   Department of Cell-Biology and Genetics
       Erasmus University
       Dr. Molenwaterplein
       NL-3015 GE Rotterdam

805   Central Laboratorium van de Bloedtransfusiedienst
       Afeling Auto-immuunziekten
       Plesmanlaan 125
       Amsterdam

Poland

806   Institute of Immunology
       Copernicus Medical School
       Cracow

807   Institute of Immunology and Experimental Therapeutics
       Polish Academy of Sciences
       Czeiska 12
       53-114 Wrocław

Scandinavia

808   Department of Immunology
       Institute of Medical Microbiology
       University of Lund
       Lund
       Sweden

809   University of Oslo
       Box 1071
       Blindern
       Oslo 3
       Norway

810   Tissue Typing Laboratory
       Rikshospitalet
       The National Hospital
       Oslo 1
       Norway

811   Department of Tumor Biology
       Karolinska Institutet 50
       S-104 01 Stockholm
       Sweden

812   Department of Immunology
       University of Umea
       Umea
       Sweden

813   Department of Immunology and the Blood Center
       University of Uppsala
       Uppsala
       Sweden

814   Departments of Medical Microbiology and Medicine
       Turku University
       Turku
       Finland

Switzerland

815   Department of Structural Biology
       Biocentre
       University of Basel
       CH-4056 Basel

816   Institute of Microbiology
       University of Basel
       Peterplatz 10
       CH-4003 Basel

817   Basel Institute of Immunology
       CH-4005 Basel 5

818   Institute of Clinical Immunology
       Inselspital
       CH-3010 Berne

819   Swiss Serum and Vaccine Institute
       Rehhagstrasse 79
       Berne

820   Institut de Biochimie
       Université de Lausanne
       Chemin des Bouveresses
       CH-1066 Epalinges

821   Department of Immunology
       Swiss Institute for Experimental Cancer Research
       CH-1066 Epalinges

822   University of Geneva
       3 Place de l'Université
       CH-1211 Geneva 4

823   WHO Immunology Research and Training Centre
       Department of Medicine
       University Hospital of Geneva
       Geneva

824   Department of Experimental Pathology
       University of Zurich
       CH-8006 Zürich

825   Institute for Immunology and Virology
       University of Zurich
       P O B
       CH-8028 Zürich

LIBRARIES — UK

SPECIALISM

826	Home Office Central Research Establishment Aldermaston Reading RG7 4PN	Forensic immunology
827	Mansion and TRD Libraries (Wellcome Labs) Langley Court Beckenham Kent BR3 3BS	General immunology
828	Veterinary Research Laboratory Northern Ireland Department of Agriculture Stormont Storey Road Belfast BT4 3SD	General and veterinary immunology
829	Beecham Pharmaceuticals Research Division Chemotherapeutic Research Centre Brockham Park Betchworth Surrey RH3 7AJ	Allergies
830	Kanthak Library Department of Pathology Cambridge University Tennis Court Road Cambridge CB2 1QP	General immunology
831	Central Veterinary Laboratory New Haw Weybridge Surrey KT15 3NB	General and veterinary immunology
832	Clinical and Population Cytogenetics Unit Western General Hospital Edinburgh EH4 2XU	Immunology and immunogenetics
833	Lister Institute of Preventive Medicine Elstree Hertfordshire WD6 3AX	Immunization and infectious diseases; Immunopathology

834	Glasgow University Library Hillhead Street Glasgow G12 8QE	General immunology
835	Glaxo Group Research Limited Greenford Road Greenford Middlesex UB6 0HE	Immunologicals
836	John Squire Medical Library Clinical Research Centre Watford Road Harrow Middlesex HA1 3UJ	Immunogenetics; Clinical immunology; Haematology; Radioisotopes
837	British Library, Science Reference Library 25 Southampton Buildings Chancery Lane London WC2A 1AW	Patent enquiries
838	Information Retrieval Limited 1 Falconberg Court London W1V 5FG	General immunology
839	Institute of Medical Laboratory Sciences 12 Queen Anne Street London W1M 0AU	Haematology; Immunology; Blood transfusion
840	Medical Research Council Library NIMR The Ridgeway Mill Hill London NW7 1AR	General immunology
841	Science Reference Library The British Library 9 Kean Street Drury Lane London WC2B 4AT	General
842	Paterson Laboratories Christie Hospital and Holt Radium Institute Wilmslow Road Manchester M20 9BX	Haematology; Immunology
843	Hoechst UK Limited Walton Manor Milton Keynes Buckinghamshire MK7 7AJ	General immunology
844	Oxford University Biochemistry Department Library South Parks Road Oxford OX1 3QU	Biochemistry; Immunology

ON-LINE DATABASE HOSTS

845 **BLAISE-Line**
The British Library
Bibliographic Services Division
2 Sheraton St
London W1V 4BH

Conference Proceedings Index
LC Marc
SIGLE
UK Marc
Whitakers

846 **BLAISE-Link**
The British Library
Bibliographic Services Division
2 Sheraton St
London W1V 4BH

AV Line
(Audiovisual catalogue
of NLM)
Cancerlit
Catline
Medline
Serline

847 **BRS**
1200 Route 7
Latham
New York 12110
USA

American Men and Women of Science
BIOSIS Previews
Books in Print
Dissertation Abstracts
Excerpta Medica
International Pharmaceutical Abstracts
IRCS Medical Science Database
MEDLARS-on-line
National Technical Information System
Pat data
Pre-Med
Predicasts Promt
Superindex
Ulrich's International

848 **Data-Star**
12 quai de la Poste
CH-1204 Geneva
Switzerland
(UK office: Willoughby Road,
Bracknell RG12 4DN,
Berkshire)

BIOSIS Previews
Cancerlit
Excerpta Medica
Medline
NTIS
Pre-Med
Predicasts Promt

849 **DIALOG**
3460 Hillview Ave
Palto Alto
California 94304
USA
(UK Office: P.O. Box 8,
Abingdon,
Oxfordshire OX13 6EG)

Book Review Index
Books in Print
Biosis Previews
CAB Abstracts
Claims
Conference Papers Index
Dissertation Abstracts Online
Embase

849 **DIALOG** (*continued*)

Federal Research in Progress
Foundation Directory
Foundation Grants Index
GPO Monthly Catalogue
International Pharmaceutical Abstracts
LC Marc
Life Sciences Collection
Medline
National Foundations
NTIS
Patlaw
PTS Promt
REMARC
Scisearch
SSIE Current Research
Telegen

850 **ESA-IRS**
Esrin
via Galileo Galilei
I-00044 Frascati
Italy

BIOSIS
CAB
Conference Papers Index

851 **OCLC**
6565 Frantz Road
Dublin
OH 43017
USA

852 **Orbit**
SDC Information Services
2500 Colorado Avenue
Santa Monica
California 90406
USA

BIOSIS
Biotechnology
Grants
LC/Line
NTIS
USPA (US Patent Office)
WPI (World Patents Index)

853 **Pergamon Infoline**
12 Vandy Street
London EC2A 2DE
England

Current awareness in the biological sciences
Inpadoc
Inpanew
Patsearch

854 **RLIN**
The Research Libraries Group Inc.
Jordan Quadrangle
Stanford
California 94305
USA

Index

All references are to page numbers. Bold-face numerals indicate a reasonably substantial entry, or the most significant of several references to a topic. Authors' names are not indexed, nor are book titles except when mentioned in the text.